"Sylvie Gouin has written a truly inspiring book. I am particularly pleased that she has made use of Yoga's stash of methods, which have so much to offer. Her advice on journaling is wise and helpful."
Georg Feuerstein, Ph.D. Author of Encyclopedia of Yoga and Tantra and 50 other books and online courses www.traditionalyogastudies.com

"Sylvie's guided journal, Inspired Living, is an excellent tool for anyone wishing to delve deeper into yogic self observation for personal and spiritual growth. We so often study yoga philosophy without taking time to integrate, to reflect on how it could change our lives. Sylvie's questions for self reflection provide a step-by-step process for examining yogic teachings through the lens of our own experience."
Chetana Panwar, Moving into Bliss with Yoga, akhandayoga.com

"I love it. LOVE it. It's perfect. It's exactly what I need (and likely, many others). It's clear, well-written, follows a natural progression and continuity, shares personal excerpts and struggles that so many of us can relate to. LOVE it. After Chapter 1, I was already inspired to set up my journaling practice. And that's why the name Inspired Living is perfect. That's what you do. That's the effect you have."
Eryn Kirkwood of Barrhaven Yoga

"Inspired Living is a unique way of learning about yogic philosophy through the heart and mind of someone who has truly studied and brought them to life in her own life decisions. Sylvie asks us to get to know ourselves through the readings, introspection and writing so that we can find choices that are supportive and that bring meaning and joy. This journal is encouraging, inspiring, and compelling. As Sylvie says in the journal, Why not try? Life is so short."
Jane Brown

"Inspired Living is a yoga journal offered to us as a clear way of getting into the awareness of our actions, our thoughts, our patterns, and all that is about each of our lives. Using the richness of yoga philosophy, and highly dedicated, experienced guidance we can tap into a world of self awareness that brings a purpose to each of us and connects us to what surrounds us. A workbook that gives us a clear understanding of how to look into what we really want to see, and how to be continuously inspired to grow to our fullest potential."
Martha Judd

Acknowledgments

Writing a guided yoga journal for personal introspection has been a dream of mine for years. This year, everything came together. I had the honor of being accepted into a mentoring program under the tutelage of Georg Feuerstein of Traditional Yoga Studies. This gave me the courage to write this journal for you, as it was confirmation that I could lead you in the right direction. In addition, my husband inspired me to take some time off from teaching, which provided me with the space to write. I am blessed to have generous friends, Martha Judd, Jane Brown, Eryn Kirkwood, and Stefania Moffatt, who kindly and generously took turns micro, and at times, macro editing. I am grateful for my daughter's interest and continuous support. Thank you to senior yoga teacher, Chetana Panwar, for taking the time to read the pre-first edition of the journal, and provide me with wise feedback for improvement. I am grateful to the many teachers and authors from whom I have studied, as well as to those who bring to life the teachings of great masters. They include Yogi Bhajan, Lynne Cardinal, Georg Feuerstein, Brenda Feuerstein, David Frawley, Marshall Govindam, Gurucharn Singh Khalsa, Marcia Solomon, Swami Vivekananda Saraswati, Pandit Rajmani Tigunait, and to the many who have made available the teachings of Ramana Maharshi, Swami Sivananda, Sri Aurobindo, and Patanjali.

Favorite Readings

I highly recommend The Deeper Dimensions of Yoga by Georg Feuerstein and Vedantic Meditations, Lighting the Flame of Awareness by David Frawley, as they are two of the most valuable books I own. It's good to have a copy of The Bhagavad Gita; my favorite translations are by Swami Sivananda and Sri Aurobindo. As for the sutras, I recommend taking the distance learning course by Traditional Yoga Studies. Some translations are challenging to integrate without a teacher, and the course leads you to greater understanding. Another option is to study privately with a local teacher. I did this with Lynne Cardinal; she helped open my eyes and led me in the right direction for personal study. I recommend books by Sri Aurobindo, and those that have been written around the teachings of Sri Ramana Maharshi.

> *To learn is to grow.*
> *To grow is to transcend.*
> *To transcend is to become free.*
> *To be free is bliss.*
> Georg Feuerstein

The Art and Science of Keeping a Spiritual Journal

The most important component to keep up with your journaling is to have your journal in sight. If you do not see it, it's easy to forget. However, we need to know that our privacy will be upheld. Take some time to consider where you could keep your journal, where you would see it every day, without it being a temptation to others.

The second key component is to keep the daily habit alive, whether it be three minutes or three hours. If you miss a few days, do not dwell, simply start over.

I encourage you to read this journal once from beginning to end without journaling. Then, begin your daily practice. How long should you journal? Everyday will provide you with different opportunities and energy levels; trust your intuition. If you don't have much time, or if you are not feeling inspired to write move to the gratitude and/or affirmation chapters, and write a few sentences.

To help organize your journal, write the full date with every entry. For example, write January 6th, 2012 as opposed to Jan 6. This will allow you to see your progress. Also, always write the page number and "for reflection" questions or the comment you are writing about. This is essential to benefit from the practice because the review process is as valuable as the act of journaling itself. There is nothing more revealing than reviewing journals from a few years past (and in some cases a few months past) to see how much we have integrated. In addition, if you keep an organized journal, you will find increased ease and willingness for this review. I highly recommend keeping a hand-written journal because you will notice your hand writing, and how it changes based on what you are writing about, and how it changes over time. Remember that this is your journal, and it lends itself to as much artistic expression as you will allow; make it your own.

If you have purchased this journal without taking the course, you may benefit from spending time with your yoga teacher to clarify a few things. If you do take the course, you will learn specific hatha yoga techniques and meditations to help further your home practice. You will find my workshop schedule at www.sylviegyoga.com; you can also contact me at 111sylvieg@gmail.com to organize a guided journal session in your area.

If you are a yoga teacher who has taken the course, and if you would like to become certified to teach Inspired Living two-hour classes, please send me three essays. The essays should include: 500 words on the philosophy presented in the text; 250 words on the benefits of keeping such a journal; 250 words on one of the golden sisters (explained in this journal.) Once everything has been reviewed, I will send you a certificate and the course outline. The cost for this is $125.00, and you can teach the course as often as you like.

Wishing you an inspired journey,

Sylvie

Will You Journal?

About 12 years ago I decided to start jogging. I was in good shape and assumed that jogging would fit right into my routine, so I decided on a 10 km jog. It turned out to be a humbling experience that left me disliking jogging. I tried a few more times but never really had a good experience. This pattern repeated itself many times over the years. I did not feel motivated enough to give this new interest the required energy—until I started running spurts when I was out hiking. I loved that. I also knew that extended travel plans would prevent me from enjoying my other sports, and regular outdoor cardiovascular exercise is not something I am willing to let go of. Therefore, I finally had meaningful reasons to give jogging another try. This time I approached it with wisdom instead of expectations. I started with short distances, and gradually increased, giving my body the time to become conditioned. When you think about it, it's not rocket science. Its patience and commitment – that's all. The same applies to our inner work. To keep up we need a reason. Some people have always been runners, it makes sense to them. I needed a reason. Journaling makes sense to me, it always has. Do you need a reason? What will it take for you to commit? Know yourself because this journal is about you, your thoughts and your beliefs, and the awareness of how they impact your experiences. What's important is to put your thoughts and beliefs on paper, and become aware of how they impact you on a daily basis and how they change over time. This type of writing brings clarity and supports introspection leading to a greater understanding of you and your life. To keep up, acknowledge that the most valuable wisdom in this journal will be your writing. Know what it will take for you to dive in, and commit.

Inspired Living: A Guided Yoga Journal

First Edition, March 2012
Copyright of Sylvie Gouin, 2012.
All Rights Reserved.

Cover design and layout by Michael Beddall

*"If you want quick spiritual attainments, you should
never neglect to record everything in your diary. The
diary is your teacher and guide. It is the eye-opener.
Blessed is he who keeps a daily diary and compares
the work of this week with that of the last week, for
he will realize quickly."*
Swami Sivananda —

About The Author

Sylvie Gouin, is a Registered Yoga Teacher ERYT500/RYT500, Registered Holistic Nutritionist and Reiki Master with over 20 years of experience. Her teaching and writing approach provides you with a balance between the guidance of a teacher and the space to have your own experiences. Her intention is simple; generously share what she has learned.

> *"The use of your writing is to keep you in touch with the inner source of inspiration and intuition so as to wear thin the crude external crust of the consciousness and encourage the growth of the inner being."*
> Sri Aurobindo

Chapter 1
The Journey 9

Chapter 2
Inspiration 13

Chapter 3
Obstacle 21

Chapter 4
Mind – Body 27

Chapter 5
The Four Golden Sisters 35

Chapter 6
The Gunas 41

Chapter 7
Ah . . . The Mind 45

Chapter 8
Equanimity 49

Chapter 9
Investment 55

Chapter 10
Morality 59

Chapter 11
The Four Aims of Life 75

Chapter 12
Gratitude 85

Chapter 13
Affirmations 87

Chapter 14
Free Flow 89

Chapter 15
Progress Report 91

Chapter 1   **The Journey**

nspired Living is a yoga journal designed for those who are interested in self exploration as a tool for growth and fulfillment. This journal functions as an inner road map, and a lifelong companion, where through review, you will get to know yourself and see and experience your own growth, and development. The end result is a personal journey that ripples out to mutual growth.

Keeping a journal is a joyful study of you. The intention is not to "get through" the study, but to take your time. Be willing to return to the beginning again and again, and review your thoughts. See and observe your progress; understanding yourself and how you relate to the world is a process valuable beyond words. As your writing unfolds, you can add pages, add questions, include the wisdom of the sages, draw pictures, or write poetry if you feel so inclined. The more you write the more you will be willing to let it unfold intuitively. Just take your time.

Remember that our experiences are often based on external factors. Our senses draw our attention outwards, impacting the thought process which then comes in contact with an emotion (either love or its opposite – a form of fear) and creates a belief. Acknowledgment that these beliefs become our truth and that many of our beliefs have been established without our paying attention is liberating. Self study asks us to pay attention, take our time and be present to our habits and life as a whole. Your journal becomes a tool that will help you become aware of the habits you have created and are creating. And, because we are creatures of habit, it's important to know what we are creating, and see that mechanical and unmindful habits built on reactions create addictions, therefore, limitations. In contrast, when we live mindfully, the habits we create are conscious choices that bring lasting joy, stamina, and overall happiness thereby nurturing a willingness—and even a desire—to pay attention. With a commitment to self study you become the light for yourself.

Through study, we train the mind to focus and we explore new territories. When we study ourselves and the scriptures, we keep up with our spiritual practice—an essential component for inspired living. Going into one's own mind and being present to the thoughts and the images that these thoughts create, as well as being present to the pulse of life, our heart beat, our breath, and our inner vibration, calms the mind's mundane activities, and gives us a taste of what we truly are after – happiness.

If we think about it, even for a short moment, we can see that, of all the things we choose to study, the conversations we engage in, the books we read, the movies and entertainment we enjoy, does it not make sense to want to know "who" is so interested, and why? Through self-observation we understand our self with honest depth. The result? We are able to make valid and life-enhancing choices

For Reflection

Ask yourself again and again, who am I? Write what comes up. Then ask, why? Where? And how did this title occur? Is it serving me? Can I let it go? Why? When? How? Ask who is asking. Try to see beyond the mind. Get to know yourself on all levels. Know your beauty, know your bliss, and know what you are sharing with the world.

My journaling journey began as a teenager reading the book, *You Can Heal Your Life* by Louise L. Hay. Hay writes that we do not have to believe everything we think. This statement had a powerful impact on me. It planted a seed that got me thinking, reading, exploring, and journaling. In the beginning, my journals were filled with intentions which, upon closer look, revealed more wants and needs than anything else. Reviewing them made me aware of this. I realized that when the mind is scattered and filled with desire, affirmations can be compared to spraying perfume in a home instead of taking the garbage out. Once I saw this pattern it became clear that the search I was calling "spiritual" was materialistically based. This is when I began, through a variety of methods, to use my journal as a tool for self observation. Over the last 25 years, I have seen shifts in myself and have gone through a variety of phases that had me investigating from different angles, most of which will be explored in this journal.

The foundation for *Inspired Living* is yogic philosophy, although no previous yoga experience is required. Yoga is a vast subject, and difficult to define, but in the context of this book I define yoga as, "an art and science of self inquiry to unravel the potential that lies within". In fact, I believe it is fair to say that self inquiry is at the heart of all yoga because yogis, like Socrates, believe that the unexamined life is not worth living. This begs the questions: what is self inquiry, and what is the art, and the science of turning inwards? The essence of self inquiry inquires into the Self capital S, which is beyond any concept we have about the Self, as well as, beyond the language we have available to us to describe "it". For example, we are often asked to meditate on the flow of the breath; to watch it move in and out. Self inquiry asks to observe: who is breathing? Who is observing?

For many, before we can take (S)elf-inquiry and internalize it with concentration, and in a manner that is beyond concept we benefit from exploring the small self. The "small s self" is a term used to describe the labels that identify this "self" we are so attached to. Clearly, when the mind is agitated, it seems impossible to sit, and truly listen. When the mind is agitated, we often do not even want to take the time to be still, and reflect deeply. As we know, we are often swayed to follow our senses, therefore, seek comfort and contentment externally. The agitation of the mind has a strong pull that keeps us identified with its habitual patterns leading us on a continuous cycle of pleasure, and pain based on expectations. Self observation leads us on an internal journey freeing us from this cycle.

The purpose of this journal is for you to study yourself with kindness and honesty. With these factors in play, you will feel yourself relax and release, thus providing mental clarity and inner peace. I created this journal to provide you with a transitional guide for your integration. As you study yourself your energy changes and this inevitably has an impact on those around you. I know too well how challenging it can be to bring this worldview to life. It's much easier to sit at home, and read about the philosophy than to implement it.

Also, I often encourage my students to journal; most smile and agree, but do not, expressing that they are unsure what to write about or the direction to take. This feedback, as well as many yoga teachers telling me that they do not use the original texts for study due to a lack of understanding, were my motivation. With dedication you will experience that keeping a journal as a tool for self exploration helps with linking thought to action, thus bringing your inner most wisdom to life.

Five main techniques will be practiced throughout this journal. They include the following:

1. **Self study:** Using the yoga *sutras* (aphorisms) of Patanjali (author of one of the most valuable yogic texts) as a foundation for reflection. These aphorisms are considered one of the world's most profound studies of the human psyche. Using the aphorisms as a foundation for self observation provides greater understanding of the mind's ingrained patterns. This observation is very cleansing, and it's much easier to set affirmations with a clean slate. The quality of affirmations change and the integration is permanent. Patanjali knew that we need to live with integrity to be able to go within, and so he placed emphasis on morality, which will also be explored in this guidebook. **Mind-Body Connection:** You will be asked to practise yoga postures, specific breathing techniques, and meditations and then relate your experiences based on specific points of focus. The list of questions provided for your practice creates an opportunity for an integrated and embodied experience;

2. **Gratitude:** One of the best expressions to open our heart, and release tension is gratitude. Gratitude is an essential component of mental clarity, thus leading to intuitive living;

3. **Focused-written affirmations** to help move beyond the mind's limiting patterns; and

4. **Progress Report:** Writing about what has changed, what has remained the same, and where and how you have grown supports an honest and clear journey.

I have no doubt that our life is part of a journey that is much bigger than we can conceptualize; journaling puts us in touch with our individuality while reminding us of what is truly important. Life is continuously unfolding and presenting itself to us, and it's easy to get caught in a whirlwind of wants, needs, worries, and complaints that keep us searching without ever feeling fulfilled. Most of us are in need of tools to awaken and *stay awake*. It takes reflection to grow beyond our current understandings, beliefs, and ingrained patterns to have genuine experiences that open our hearts and expand our minds. My hope is that this journal will lead the way, and as your writing shifts and unveils your intuition, you will see your light shine through. As the saying goes: "The journey of a thousand miles begins with one step, and that one step must be from where you stand."

It's important to acknowledge that keeping a journal is a spiritual, and sacred practice, requiring mindful, and benevolent attention. Do you have space at home for your introspection? If not, create it. Create an inviting and well-lit space for yourself. There is no need to go shopping to prepare the space; simplicity is often best. Remove clutter, ensure that you can sit comfortably, and that the environment feels supportive of your writing. I always journal with colored gel pens. I like the feel and the look of them. What do you like? Take some time and think it through for yourself.

As a sacred practice, creating a ritual sets the mood. Plato tells us that "the beginning is the most important of any work". Make a good beginning for yourself. Communicate, light incense and/or a candle, play supportive music, set your intention, chant, pray, or simply take a few minutes before you start writing to close your eyes and take some slow, deep breaths.

My ritual looks like this: I close my eyes, take a few deep breaths, get comfortable, go within, and remind myself of my intention for journaling. The reminder at this point is not through words; it's a feeling. I chant my mantra, and then verbally communicate something along these lines: "God be in my mind and in my heart. Bless me with the ability to hear my inner wisdom and trust my intuition. May my study prove to be liberating. I am eternally grateful for the wisdom shared by so many teachers." I then thank a few people who have influenced me. Who I thank is intuitive and changes.

For Reflection
Ask yourself, what kind of ritual are you willing to commit to? To help with this reflection, look at what hobbies or ways of being currently give you energy when you do them and that leave you feeling less than par when you do not? What is important is that the ritual you create be meaningful to you.

You can write your ritual down, or let it be intuitive, depending on your personality. Your ritual may change over time. Just know that as long as it's heartfelt, and honest, it will create the right energy.

"Happiness is your nature. It is not wrong to desire it.
What is wrong is seeking it outside when it is inside."
Sri Ramana Maharshi

Chapter 2   **Inspiration**

M ost of the yoga styles we see today are variations of Hindu-based yoga. Hinduism is a spiritual tradition that accepts all useful practices towards individual freedom or enlightenment which is the central purpose of Hindu-based yoga. The accurate name for Hinduism is *Sanatana Dharma*, meaning "eternal truth". Know that Hinduism does not emphasize a book, a prophet, or a church. It's a living unfolding of eternal truth, which accepts and flows with the natural changes in human conditions. Therefore, to practice Hindu-based yoga you need not change religions or belief systems.

Regarding spirituality, in this regard it's about bringing to life the perfection of your individuality as an interconnected source. The more we become acquainted with our individuality through self introspection, the more we realize the impact morality plays on our life. Yogis have always made it an integral aspect of spirituality because morality leads our everyday life. Our judgment of what is good and bad affects our behavior, and thus, our state of mind. Just like a dirty, cluttered, noisy home makes it challenging to be introspective, so does a mind filled with greed, anger, jealousy, and resentment. Ingrained in the teachings is the reminder that morality is at the core of what keeps us human, of what keeps us conscious. Morality is of the utmost importance to the yogi in large part because our thoughts and actions leave karmic imprints. It's hard to disagree with the theory that we are not only a product of our past experiences, but also of how we relate to them. Yoga masters have been teaching us for thousands of years that immoral actions lead to suffering and pain, and moral actions put forth without attachments reduce mental agitation, thereby increasing the potential for enlightenment. This journal will ask you to reflect on certain aspects of your life and, through introspection, will help you to establish your own centre of balance in support of your spiritual expression.

As a new student of yoga I found myself seeking answers in many different places. On one hand, I benefited from that process, but on the other hand, I was left with even more confusion. Often when going to a talk, retreat, workshop, or even when reading a book, we are not necessarily told from which perspective the teacher, author, or master is speaking and there are many perspectives in the world of yoga. I was not aware of it at the time, but what I wanted was clear answers to what yoga is; what yoga believes is; and the only possible method for liberation is.

I finally had to accept that the yogic tradition is rich in wisdom, and to grasp even a small fraction of it requires tremendous dedication. In today's world, we have access to so much information that it's not uncommon to take a little from here and a little from there, thus creating a variety of modern-day yoga schools of thought. I remember at times feeling overwhelmed by the vastness, and the richness of the philosophy. My desire to know it all left me feeling intimidated by what I did not know and would probably not know or be able to practice, for that matter. I remember times sitting for meditation not knowing which of the many methods I should use!

Throughout this exploration I never saw myself as a seeker, as someone looking to know it all. However, as soon as I stopped searching I saw it clearly. No doubt the experience was what I needed, and the knowledge I collected had a lasting effect on me. Still, the best thing I ever did to integrate all of these teachings was to stop and reflect on why I chose to practice. I asked myself: what is it that I want? And where is it that I am trying to get? These questions provided me with respite from my external search for the ultimate wisdom that leads to inner freedom. Furthermore, stopping – really stopping – allowed me to feel the vibration of my body. I then realized that to integrate and to have an experience, I needed to calm down.

For Reflection
What do I want? Why? What am I trying to achieve? Why?

Over the years, I created a variety of journals, asking all sorts of questions of what I felt was valuable, and which aspects of this great tradition I could or would actually put into practice. I had to be fully honest. It's one thing to dream of awakening, and then providing that awakening for others, but it's another to implement the amount of dedication and discipline that this requires. It takes work, and for me, the type of work that it takes is often done in silence. I eventually came to realize that there is one yoga and one method that leads to liberation: it's the one that I practice.

The following seven reflections are significant to support your quest and integrate the teachings in your daily life. Take your time with them and always remember that this process is not a race.

For Reflection
1. Ask yourself what you hope to gain from your yoga, journaling or other spiritual practice, and choose the authors and teachers you want to learn from accordingly;

2. Know what is available in terms of spiritual practices, and ask yourself what you can commit to with concentration and benevolence, and set your goals accordingly. For example: "I will journal every day, I will meditate, and practice 20 minutes of yoga every morning.";

3. Ask yourself if you can you commit to a generous, and compassionate attitude through your thoughts, words and action. Can you value where you are, who you are with, and life itself as it is? Why? How?;

4. Know what type of attitude and actions are required to nourish patience, and fuel it daily. Be aware of how patience and impatience manifests in you, and in those around you. See clearly the value of nourishing this beautiful quality and give it space to blossom;

5. Remember that getting to know yourself and listening to the voice of intuition is more valuable than trying to learn as much as you can about everything spiritual;

6. Open your eyes to see and feel the beauty of nature in all of its aspects. Give yourself some ideas on how to consciously interact with Mother Nature; and

7. Learn to listen. Listen to your thoughts, your breath, your words and your tone of voice. Learn to listen to those around you with all of your senses. Do you currently see yourself as a good listener? Why? Be open to improving on your ability to understand others and hear what they are saying.

Review these points often and adjust as needed; make them yours.

The following is a brief description of Hindu-based yoga, the foundation for this journal. I include it as a base of understanding of the philosophy provided for your introspection. Before we explore the different schools let us clarify a few terms.

Hinduism is rooted in the *vedas*. *Vedic* traditions are ancient, and rich in differential philosophies including dualistic (*dvaita*), and nondualistic (*advaita*) vedantic world views. Dvaita philosophy recognizes the essence of who we are as pure, and untouched by nature. This philosophy refers to this aspect of our Self as *jiva* or *purusha* (spirit or soul) as separate from Ishwara, the supreme God. *Advaita* philosophy looks at everything as Brahman, the supreme God. And in this case Brahman includes the essence of who we are. In *advaita vedanta* we must experience, and realize the unity of everything to achieve our full potential. Until we achieve our full potential, *advaita vedanta* uses the system of duality to explain our relationship to consciousness, matter, and how there is a direct split between the two. Simply put, *dvaita* considers the *jiva* eternal, but dependent upon God, never equal. *Advaita* believes that the experience of *sat chit ananda* (existence-consciousness-bliss) is the expression of God.

Schools of Hindu-Based Yoga:

Bhakti Yoga: This devotional yoga approach is referred to extensively in the *Bhagavad-Gita* (a sacred text of 700 verses, considered to be one of the most important works of Hindu philosophy). Representing the relationship between the student and the divine, bhakti yoga provides the householder with a clear path to living with awareness in this world. With the belief that the divine is in all, and is present at every moment, this path teaches us to treat everyone with kindness and benevolence. *Bhakti* is not only a path of devotion for devotion, but is a path of devotion towards liberation.

Hatha Yoga: Hatha yoga is a form of *tantra* yoga (to weave), and the foundation of most of today's popular yoga styles. The word *hatha* is often translated as sun and moon, but it really means two opposing energies. The word hatha itself means force. The three main texts for hatha yoga are the *Hatha Yoga Pradipika*, the *Gheranda-Samhita*, and the *Shiva Samhita*. The *Hatha Yoga Pradipika*, was written by the sage Swatmarama in the 14th century and consists of 389 stanzas organized into four chapters. This book discusses and describes cleansing practices, postures, breath control, seals, and the importance of awakening the *kundalini* energy. The *Gheranda-Samhita* is said to have been composed at the end of the 17th century.

In it, the path of hatha yoga is described as being sevenfold, including cleansing techniques, postures, seals, sensory inhibition, breath control, meditation, and ecstasy. The third text, The *Shiva Samhita*, is considered the most comprehensive treatise of hatha yoga (believed to be written in the 17th or 18th century). This text has a distinct Buddhist influence, it discusses liberation and describes 84 postures, only four of which are said to be important. Although many more ancient texts of hatha yoga have been written, most of them are difficult to attain, and impossible to understand without deep inner practice, and a realized teacher.

Karma Yoga: *Karma* means action, and refers to every action we have ever done, including those that occurred in our past lives. *Karma* explains how these actions affect our present circumstances. A karma yogi dedicates every action as an offering to the divine. In short, *karma* yoga is right action in accordance with the laws of *dharma* (your unique path).

Jnana Yoga: *Jnana*, the path of wisdom, is nondualist, and is the path of the vedanta tradition. Jnana yoga believes in living liberation, and considers transcendental reality as the self, here and now. One of the leading authorities on jnana yoga, Ramana Maharshi (1879-1950), recommended the practice by which he experienced his enlightenment, a practice where the aspirant is to ponder the question, who am I? This is a *vedantic* approach, where we answer "*neti-neti*" (not thus not thus) to the mind's association to the question. It's combined with a deep inner listening, and awareness of inner silence that allows the veils of distraction, and identification to fade away, allowing us to experience our true self.

Mantra Yoga: The practice of mantra yoga is an art, and a science, where the student focuses on the vibration of each letter of the Sanskrit alphabet, and on the vibrations of the words created by them. Mantra yoga describes sound as a vehicle for transcendence. The discovery that repetitive sound affects consciousness was made long ago, perhaps as early as the Stone Age. Therefore, by the time of Vedic civilization, sound was a sophisticated means of expression. Sound as a means for conscious growth, devotion, and elevation has since become a part of our world, and of many traditions. The word mantra has its roots in *manas* (mind) and *trana* (saving). A mantra is that which saves the mind from itself. It is a sacred utterance charged with psychospiritual powers.

Raja (Royal) Yoga: Royal yoga refers to Patanjali's popular eight-fold path of ethical living, practice, and meditation, which is largely the foundation for this journal.

Most of the original texts supporting this worldview are written in Sanskrit, a beautiful and ancient Vedic language. Sanskrit means perfect, pure, or polished and is the language you may not recognize in this journal. To help identify it, I always italicize it. The study of this language is mantra yoga. Most of the texts we read have been translated from Sanskrit by a variety of scholars and yogis; this is one of the reasons we see varying beliefs and practices.

A Little Bit About Yoga and God

Many moons ago when I taught yoga classes in schools, I was invited to teach in a Catholic school. Most parents and the Catholic school faculty were welcoming, and happy to have the service available for their children, except for one parent who was appalled. He felt that yoga and Hinduism go hand-in-hand, and worried about what I was going to teach the children. What really surprised me was the response from the school board and the other parents. They felt that his reaction was inappropriate, and were certain that there is nothing religious or godly about yoga. Sometimes it seems the more popular something gets the more we lose its true essence. We pick and choose what we like about a tradition, or a methodology, and leave behind what does not suit us. It's much like peeling an apple and throwing out the core. We run the risk of getting rid of too much, and in the end, we shortchange ourselves.

As you know, the appalled parent was indeed correct. Yoga is influenced by Hinduism, but Buddhist, Jains and Sikhs also have their yoga. And the beliefs, and practices vary substantially. Some yogis believe in God and others do not. In addition, many Hindu-based hatha yoga teachers practice Buddhist-based meditation, and although Buddhism, and Hinduism share common ground, such as the search for enlightenment, the belief in reincarnation, and the belief that the student needs a teacher, the scriptures, and a community of like-minded people to grow, when it comes to God, the commonalities end.

The foundation of this journal finds its roots in the three following texts, and God is at the heart of them all:

1. **Bhagavad-Gita** is one of the pillars of Hindu bhakti yoga, and is based on non-dualistic *vedanta*. *Bhagavad-Gita* presents 18 chapters, each can be said to be a yoga, and all set out three main paths for ultimate union with God. One of the central teachings is to live one's unique duty, and purpose without attachment to results. It's a wise, and supportive read for anyone who values living with benevolent equanimity;

2. **Yoga Sutras of Patanjali** is a unique philosophic worldview, which unlike most teachings, moves beyond philosophy to provide us with a method for self transformation. *The Yoga Sutras of Patanjali* describes the subtle experience of each stage of mindfulness, from how to move beyond gross obstacles to the most advanced aspects of oneness.

It's fair to say that Patanjali is to yoga what Buddha is to Buddhism. The goal of the teachings is the same: to end suffering. We do this by realizing that we contribute to our own suffering through lack of mindfulness. By understanding how the mind works, and transcending its tendencies, the Self (as opposed to the "self") shines and leads the way. The *sutras* (thread) of Patanjali are a compilation of 196 aphorisms separated in four distinctive chapters. In *sutra* 2.1 we find that burning zeal in practice, self study, and study of the scriptures, as well as surrender to God are the acts of yoga. This *sutra* is the foundation for a yogic approach to healthy (established in the self) living. Also know that when Patanjali describes the obstacles on our spiritual path he also provides us with a few techniques to move beyond the obstacles and includes sutra 1.39, which is persistent meditation in accordance/harmony to our religious heritage; and

3. **The Hatha-Yoga Pradipika:** *Pradipika* is a Sanskrit verb defined as "to flame forth"; that is, to bring light to a subject, and in this case, a light that also brings clarity. It's a book full of metaphors and analogies, designed for those who are ready to dedicate the time to practice and therefore, understanding. There is no doubt that it's an esoteric work that requires empirical research with a teacher, in a supportive environment. This text teaches that the highest purpose of life is becoming one with God.

Based on these three texts we can see that God realization is definitely at the heart of Hindu-based yoga. But what is meant by God?

Depending on the school of thought, God can be seen as the energy of awareness, not necessarily a personal God. Also, Patanjali describes Ishwara (God) as being beyond time, and the teacher of the earliest teachers. Some yogis describe God as the Witness of the Witness, as Pure Consciousness, or Pure Awareness.

The beauty of this is that, with a little guidance, and reflection, you can choose your path and can practice yoga authentically. Know that when the name of God is mentioned it's "your God". You see, in the end, this *philo* (love) *sophy* (wisdom) is not interested in whether you believe in God or not. What's important is how your belief impacts your life, and the life of others. In short, does your belief open or close your heart?

Always remember that your practice is working for you if you see yourself opening up mentally and physically. If you become more rigid and unnecessarily judgmental, something is not flowing.

Therefore, if you practice with awareness, respect, curiosity, and dedication, yoga will be of service to you and will ripple out in your everyday living.

For Reflection

Do I believe in God? Who is it that I believe in or don't believe in? How does this sit in my heart? How does it serve me? Where did this belief come from? How does it impact my life? Is there a possibility that I could approach my belief from a different perspective? If yes, what would that look like? If not, why not?

I have pondered these questions silently, and I also pondered these questions with a pen and paper. The more I answer and write, the more questions arise; at some point I intuitively stop. These writings stimulate my mind, open my heart, and impact my energy when I sit in meditation as well as in my everyday life. I love rereading and watching my own unfolding, which reveals fewer and fewer words. Take your time. Write the above mentioned questions, and reflect. See what arises for you.

> *"Society is the product of relationship, of yours and mine together. If we change in our relationship, society changes."*
>
> J. Krishnamurti

Chapter 3

Obstacles

I have been educating my daughter about managing her finances since she was quite young. At 18, she now has an understanding of how to create stability and prosperity for herself. Recently, she sent me an email explaining that she was overspending, and felt discouraged by her habit. I told her to start her budget again, right now. Stop reflecting on what you feel has been a failure, and return to your intentions. I also reminded her that if it was easy to be so well-organized financially, our world would be a different place. See the pattern in yourself and start over. Do not dwell! Accept that it takes work. The same is true of our introspective path. Regardless of your surroundings or starting points, you undoubtedly will encounter obstacles. I am advising you in the same manner. Do not dwell, see it, move beyond it, and remember if it was easy, would our world be as it is?

To help guide us, Patanjali lists in *sutra* 1.30 the nine possible obstacles as: sickness; languor; doubt; heedlessness; sloth; dissipation; false view; non-attaining of the stages; and instability. *sutra* 1.31, lists what accompanies these obstacles: pain; depression; tremor of the limbs; wrong inhalation; and exhalation.

Let us look at each of these obstacles in more detail.

1. **Sickness:** As we all know, when the body is sick it's very difficult to focus on anything else. Being born healthy is quite the gift, and yet many people take it for granted, filling the body and the mind with all sorts of junk food and junk information that takes away from the vitality of the body and mind.

For Reflection

How do you define health? How do you define sickness? Do you consider yourself a healthy person? One of the Sanskrit words for health is *swastha* and it means to be established in the Self. Does that statement mean anything to you? Do you see yourself as someone who is established in the Self? In the English language wholeness is the etymology for the words health, integrity and integration. What does wholeness mean to you?

Sickness and disease go hand-in-hand and if we take the word disease and divide it, we read "dis" and "ease". Therefore, we can see that disease is defined as being without "ease". How would you define being at ease? Are you at ease?

When you are sick, what kind of energy do you feed? Are you dramatic? Do you feel pity for yourself? Do you ignore it? How are you with those you love when they are sick? Some of us set very high expectations and experience a sense of failure when we are sick. Do you see yourself here? Do you express gratitude for your health? Are you able to learn and find your centre of balance when you are ill or in pain?

Here is a personal example of how I used a health issue to move beyond a reactive state of mind. I had a skin irritation that made me itch everywhere. Scratching would not help, it would simply aggravate. I thought of people going through major health crises and remembered that I too may at some point experience a deeper health issue. Would I be able to respond? Would I react? I chose to use this mild experience and build stamina; I avoided scratching, took some deep breaths, and moved beyond it.

Write about your personal experiences.

2. **Languor:** Weakness of body and mind. Very few people want to claim weakness as it's the type of energy that lends itself to failure.

For Reflection

How do you define weakness of mind? How do you define weakness of body? How do you define strength of mind? How do you define strength of body? Do you see yourself as being at risk for weakness? If so, how can you move beyond it?

3. **Doubt:** A little voice in the back of your mind questioning everything, doubt can be your friend or your enemy. Healthy doubt motivates you to keep up and find the answers for yourself. Negative doubt feeds the ego, and suppresses your energy levels.

For example, as you progress on your path of self observation, you may at times doubt a methodology, or doubt your ability to follow through with your initial commitment. As we know, it's not uncommon to doubt things, thus choose not to try the method instead of doubting the method and putting it into practice to gain our own experience. Know that yogis want you to approach the path like a scientist. They want you to question and experience the benefits of the practice first hand. They want you to use doubt in your favor. Doubt will only be an obstacle if you allow it to limit your potential for unique experiences.

Question, listen, and practice. If you are questioning your ability for self discipline, move beyond it. The ability to move beyond this limitation is often associated with the fear of letting go of what we know and the belief, as David Frawley explains in *Lighting the Flame of Awareness*, that we believe we are afraid of the unknown when what we are actually afraid of, is what we know we don't like, or what we think we know we do not like of what we do know.

For Reflection

Be aware of how doubt works in your life. Notice when you feel more doubtful and when you are willing to accept the information given. How does doubt currently impact your life? Over the next few days, be present and see what arises for you. Sri Ramana Maharshi reminds us that doubt will always be an obstacle unless we can establish a relationship with "who" is doubting. Keep reflecting on this "who" in your journal, by asking who believes this? What is the source of this belief?

4. **Heedlessness:** Heedlessness can be defined as to be thoughtless, and careless. It's a lack of mindfulness, and awareness. Like most things spoken of, this is not black and white. Most of us come in and out of heedlessness and heedful behaviors. They are both on a scale of some sort. I am sure that some of us are considered heedless in certain situations and know in our heart that it could be better, that with discipline and concentration we could move forward. Yet we also see that we are heedful in other circumstances.

For Reflection

How can you provide close and meaningful attention to your practice and to your life? Take some time, and reflect on where heedlessness manifests in your day. What types of qualities could you nurture to move beyond it? When are you heedful? How does it manifest?

5. **Sloth:** Defined as spiritual apathy. In Christianity, it's one of the seven deadly sins as it can destroy our ability for empathy, and compassion. Sloth (laziness) has a heavy energy, and the heavier we feel, the deeper we sink, and the harder it seems to get up. Never forget that getting started can be the most difficult thing; once started you will not stop because you will remember how difficult it can be to start again. Do not allow sloth to settle in, keep up with your practice, and be vigilant.

For Reflection

Would you consider yourself at risk for sloth? Is this something you need to pay attention to? If so, what will you do to avoid its downfall? How will you see it in yourself?

6. **Dissipation:** Too much focus on feeding the needs of the body (sleep, food, sex) creates no *tapas* (internal fire explored in more detail in chapter 10), just lavish excess.

For Reflection

Do you see yourself as being easily swayed by the senses? Are you always looking for sense gratification? How does this serve you? Do you believe in being moderate? Why? How does this belief impact you and the decisions you make? Are you at risk for extremes?

7. **False Vision:** Delusions and misunderstandings create confusion of what should, or could be attained, and leaves us feeling unsettled.

For Reflection

Do you have expectations of your practice? What are they? Why? Can you let them go? When? How

8. **Non-attaining of the Stages:** Expectations of what and when stages should be experienced leads to depression, resentment, and distraction. Our mind is busy, and it creates all sorts of expectations for us to fulfill; we then use the same distracted aspect of the mind to evaluate our results. This results when we focus heavily on our expectations of "more advanced stages" rather than allowing them to unravel as true nature.

In some cases, the spiritual practice becomes more about being "in" than it does about going within. Over the years, I have met many people, and have seen how the practice progressed in different surroundings. The following example will help define what I want to express. To help guide my writing, I use the journey of an acquaintance. Let us call my yogini Chantal. Chantal begins yoga, takes one class and falls in love. She keeps returning to class as often as she can. She expresses that she feels a deep sense of connection with the practice. Within about one year, she signs up for yoga teacher training and within two years, she quits her profession to pursue teaching yoga full time. In another four years Chantal has not only stopped teaching yoga, but has also stopped practicing. She says, "I had enough of the scene. If I practice now it is just a bit of stretching at home."

The fact that someone who felt so connected to the practice can relate to yoga as "a bit of stretching", tells me that sometimes we want something so badly we convince ourselves we have tasted its nectar when really we have fallen in love with the idea of what we think we want. This is why introspection is so important. Do not allow yourself to live a lie; you can tap into the deeper aspects of yoga. The benefits of the practice are real. However, we get out of it what we put into it. It's always a balance of keeping up, and letting go of expectations.

For Reflection

Stages of yoga; what does that mean to you? How would you define this? Where do you see yourself? Do you have expectations of where you should be? Are you there? Why? How? Can you let your expectations go? Why? How? When?

9. **Instability:** Refers to an inability to stay with the task at hand, and is a result of a scattered mind, body, and life expression. From this perspective, Patanjali speaks of our inability to keep the aspect of the mind that is always in movement in focus. Anyone who has tried to do this is aware of the challenges this poses. We need to focus and be present, train our minds to work in our favor. Know that

creating external stability will help establish a relationship with this energy. Nourishing the ability to find your centre in your everyday life regardless of what arises brings mental clarity. Start with small things, cultivate the habit, and feed the energy with benevolence. Eventually we will be able to remain stable when the external is chaotic, but we benefit from the reverse to breathe in the energy fully.

For Reflection

How do you see stability? How do you see instability? Are you able to focus? For how long? What draws your attention? Why? How does instability manifest? How can you cultivate focus in your life?

Being aware of the obstacles is key as it helps to see them as we live them as opposed to live them as our truth, and identify with them. If we can see the experience, we are not "it". This understanding is something very tangible, and an accessible experience to stay focused, or nurture the ability to focus. As you go through this journal, you will learn, and begin to integrate more and more lifestyle choices that sustain vitality, allowing you to move beyond these obstacles. Keeping a journal makes us aware of the brilliance that lies within. As it unfolds, the desires that keep us stuck melt away. In my experience, I have not woken up suddenly, and relinquished my human aspirations, but I no longer feel defined by my success, or failure as I used to, and I do experience a deep sense of acceptance as I grow, integrate, learn, and start over.

Our habits can be so deeply engrained that we may hold onto them, even when they bring discomfort and pain. Exploring your true nature will inevitably result in your letting go of some things you currently think you love. I am here to reassure you that the path when practised authentically unfolds brilliantly. Yes, you will encounter some discomforts, some growing pains, but eventually it settles and you start to experience inner stability and contentment, even as you go through the challenging times. Yoga is not about creating more wants and needs, even if the needs transform from new shoes to inner bliss.

For Reflection

Take some time and write about these obstacles. How do you relate to them as a whole? Does it make sense to you? Do you agree with Patanjali? Why? Can you see the potential for the obstacles to create a barrier with your willingness for a deeper understanding of yourself and life as a whole? Does knowing about them bring clarity, therefore, potential to move beyond them?

In addition to listing the obstacles, Patanjali provides us with antidotes to move beyond them. Some of these antidotes will be explored throughout this journal.

"Breathe - Smile - Believe"

Chapter 4

Mind Body Connection
Hatha Yoga: The Practice

As mentioned, hatha yoga is concerned with the awakening of *kundalini* energy. *Kundalini,* defined as "she who is coiled" is a powerful energy residing in every cell of our being, patiently waiting to be awakened through its union with *prana* (life force). The word *kundalini* finds its root in the word *kunda,* meaning fire pit. *Anda* is a self-contained egg that is saturated with the very principle of creativity. *Kundalini shakti* is the power that resides in this fire pit. What makes the kundalini experience so unique is that it not only creates a transcending mental experience, but it also includes the physical body.

When I began my yoga journey, *kundalini* was what caught my attention. I loved the word *kundalini,* and the image of *kundalini* awakening and leading me beyond my perceptions to ultimate freedom was enough to keep me inspired and motivated. Although I realize I did not have a real understanding of what was meant by *kundalini,* my imagined ideas kept me disciplined and committed. Clearly, our perceptions and understandings are always what we have. As verse 60 of the 4th chapter of the *Hatha Yoga Pradipika* reminds us: "All of this world, animate and inanimate, is the appearance of mind." In retrospect, I can see that my connection was based on illusory fantasies, and I think that people who are at that stage of understanding are often attracted to these aspects based on magical beliefs. Our mind follows the animation it creates. This can cause problems as we may identify with the desire and somehow fuel ourselves this way. If someone is of a more rational nature and hears people speak of such things, they may relate the whole esoteric aspect of yoga to this fantasy. We are all trying to define experiences with a limited language, and there is nothing "magical" about kundalini. To believe so and be limited by this belief would be like saying that water is evil because of the tsunami. We must have our own experience, and we can only have it through practice. Without practice, kundalini awakening either makes no sense, or we may try and make sense out of it by inventing experiences and convincing ourselves to believe our lies. We must move beyond both these options and gain our own experience by always keeping up with our spiritual practices and by always letting go of expectations.

For Reflection

Do you ever feel weighed down by the memories you are choosing to entertain over and over again? Do you invent images of what could happen
based on those memories? Do you ever miss the beauty that lies in front
of you because you were lost in thought? How does this serve you? How
can you develop the opposite?

There is no denying that what we focus on grows, and that our perceptions shape
and dictate our experiences. We always see the world, our world, based on the angle
we are using. Perspectives determine the memories we have and therefore much of
our behavior. If you have a physical therapist, an architect and a business owner
walking down the same street, they will most likely notice different things as they
make their way to their destination. The physical therapist notices peoples' postures,
the architect sees the buildings, and the business owner notices the businesses.

As we age and gain new experiences, what we take in also changes. As a child walking into a candy store, cavities and blood sugar are not on your mind, but as a mother, the candy store is not as attractive. When we are willing to admit the limitations
that this creates, we start to open up and see and experience life with more depth.
Recognizing fully that we see what we see based on what we value, and that when
we value something, we give it life reminds us to pay attention to what matters.

One of my favorite definitions of the ripple effect of an awakened yoga practice is
that we start to breathe life into our everyday life.

The following is a short list of the signs that your kundalini is awakening:

1. An interest in this work and philosophy;
2. A continuous increase of the virtue of patience;
3. A balanced increase in physical, mental, and emotional endurance and stamina;
4. Integrated mental clarity;
5. You take responsibility for your thoughts, words, and actions;
6. You are no longer led by the senses or looking outside yourself for stimulation,
   but instead are the master of yourself;
7. You have the ability to clearly see, and discern between what is useful within you,
   and fully able to let go without attachment, or pride to what is detrimental and
   useless; and
8. You are capable to restrain yourself, and live with discipline joyfully and content.

The following are techniques that support the awakening of kundalini:

1. Offer great respect for divinity;
2. Open your heart and nourish a curious, and sattvic mind. (explored in chapter 6);
3. Practice hatha yoga; it strengthens the body, and balances the nervous system,
   creating the right environment for increasing energy;

4. Focus on the *manipura chakra* (a technique described later in this text) to generate the heat, and necessary power to awaken your *kundalini* energy;

5. *Pranayama* (breathing practices) to balance the nervous system, and assist in creating, and sustaining a calm, and clear mind. This calm mind is a catalyst to direct itself in the right direction. As mentioned, without this direction, the mind is often preoccupied with the stimulation from the external world, which it receives from the senses, thus preventing internal focus. Regular *pranayama* practices have the potential to channel the *pranic* energy, and eventually awaken *kundalini*;

6. Concentrate and meditate on the *chakras*. This practice helps to shift consciousness from the body, and its physical functions to an inner state;

7. Philosophical study of the self, and of the scriptures, which is what this journal provides; and

8. Devotion to God, to sound, to nature, and to life itself.

Now, let's look at how to bring these techniques to life. We will begin with the practice of yoga *asanas* and *pranayamas*. Practising hatha yoga *asana* in your everyday life can be as simple as being aware of your posture. Noticing how we stand and how we hold our self is highly valuable in our relationships as so much of what we say is through our body language.

In addition, we must acknowledge that a good posture is the foundation of a hatha yoga practice. Without it, we bring our poor posture to every other yoga posture, thus increasing our potential for injury. Even if you already have an excellent posture, spend the next week paying attention to how you hold yourself in different situations, notice how others hold themselves and the image and messages you receive from them. Write a few words about what you notice.

Practising the following consciously and regularly will help you establish excellent posture even when you are not thinking about it:

- Stand with your feet hips width apart;
- Feet straight;
- Weight evenly distributed on each foot;
- Balls of the feet and heels evenly grounded;
- Knees straight;
- Legs engaged;
- Hips neutral;
- Thoracic spine coming towards the chest;
- Chest lifting slightly;
- Scapula' (shoulder blades) move downwards - away from the ears;
- Chin slightly tucked in;
- Earlobes in line with the centre of the shoulders;

- Soften your mental edge and smile; and
- As you inhale ground the legs, as you exhale feel the upper body rising. Repeat three to five times.

I highly encourage you to speak with your yoga teacher or with a fitness expert for an individual postural assessment. This is valuable regardless of how long we have been practising or teaching. There is so much value in allowing attentive, intelligent and kind eyes to help us see what we cannot see on our own.

Benefits of improving your posture include:
- Increases positive attitude;
- Nurtures self confidence;
- Improves digestion;
- Increases overall energy;
- Reduces unnecessary physical discomforts;
- Tones the abdominal muscles;
- Aligns the spine and prevents wearing of the joints; and
- Improves appearance.

These are just a few of the benefits. As you can see there is so much value in being aware of our posture. In addition, becoming aware of how you hold yourself and making an effort to stand tall will provide space for your diaphragm, the primary muscle of respiration, to move with ease, thus releasing holding patterns. Adding conscious breathing will bring an overall sense of well being. Dr. Weil, a graduate of Harvard Medical School and author of nine books on the mind-body connection is quoted as saying: "If I had to limit my advice on healthier living to just one tip, it would be simply to learn how to breathe correctly." This is a powerful statement, and so true.

Recognizing the profound connection between the nervous system, and the respiratory system will encourage you to breathe consciously. Again, imagine feeling mentally clear and able to focus. This is our true nature; we just need some help to maintain it, not because it's unnatural but because our social conditioning and way of life is unnatural. Awareness of the breath helps establish and maintain a positive attitude and sustains our energy.

Be conscious of your starting point. It's not uncommon to become a chest breather, creating shallow breaths and impacting the body as a whole. The diaphragm, located below the ribcage, is meant to move downward when we inhale, creating an expansion (not a bloating) of the abdomen. If you have been breathing shallow breaths for many years, it will take time to reconnect with proper breathing. The diaphragm, also being a muscle, atrophies if it's not used. It takes practice to rebuild strength and vitality. With patience and concentration it will return.

The body wants to be healthy, wants to return to balance. Let the mind be of service to it. Regardless of where you are on your path, it's always a good idea to sit privately with a senior yoga teacher and explore the breath. I ask you to remain a beginner and even if you have years of practice behind you, pay attention, as it's also not uncommon to over breathe at some point on our journey.

I remember when I started my practice and we had to sit still, and breathe. I thought I would go out of mind. I didn't have the patience to slow my breath down, and watch it. Even today, when I am going through difficult situations and feel some anxiety, sitting, and breathing deeply is challenging. I want to rush through the breath, and move on. Take care of what needs to be done. What I notice, is that if I do spend the time breathing, a couple of things happen: either I realize that what I was stressed about was not as big as I thought, or the mental clarity from calming down helps me establish a better relationship with the solution.

This week, be very conscious of your breath in different situations. Notice how when you breathe, the people around you start to breathe. You don't need to stop doing what you are doing; you can breathe deeply anytime, anywhere. Find your natural rhythm, not through force, but through awareness. Write about your experiences.

Let us further our relationship with the breath with the regular practice of *nadi-shod-hanam* (alternate nostril breathing), one of the most beneficial practices to balance the nervous system, and eliminate impurities (please take the time to learn this from a qualified teacher).

How To:

Sit tall, and relaxed as taught in class, or from your teacher. Place your left hand on your knee with your fingers in *guyan mudra*, (thumb and index finger touching with palm up or down), and place your right hand in *vishnu mudra* (index and middle finger tucked in). Block the right nostril with the right thumb. Remember to block high up on the nose, were the nostril starts to open up. Ensure that you have exhaled fully before beginning. To begin, inhale slowly through the left nostril, then block the left nostril with the fingers of the right hand, lift the thumb and exhale right. Continue by inhaling right and exhaling left slowly then repeat the pattern. Close by exhaling fully through the left nostril.

How many times? Start with a commitment you can maintain. I recommend eight slow full rounds daily for the next 120 days. Eventually you will want to increase the time.

There is one issue with this practice. You see, to reap the benefits you need to practice.

For Reflection

Will I practice? Think of the obstacles, which ones may interfere? How do you plan on staying committed and move beyond the potential obstacles? Write about what arises for you.

As for your *asana* practice (if you do not have a regular practice it's never too late to start or start again), the following journaling inquiries will help you gain wisdom with your mind-body connection. To understand *asana* know that there are two roots to the word asana. One means "a good seat" for the body and the mind, and the other means "to be". The following may sound like a platitude, but we are human beings, not human doings. Therefore, it's impossible to "do" yoga; you can only "be" yoga. This awareness awakens our consciousness, letting the small ego, the one who likes to compare herself with others, rest for a while, and helps us practice with wisdom.

Bring the following inquiries (one at a time of course) to your *asana* practice (class.) Remember to write about what you remember arising within you. Writing really is more revealing than keeping it in your head.

Notice the following:

- Are you fully committed to your asana practice? What does that mean? Why?;
- How do you move in and out of postures? Sometimes we rush out, or rush in, possibly ignoring the process. Write what really occurred and write your aspirations. Then give yourself the permission to see the perfection of where you are and what you are experiencing because this is where we find the true experience of yoga. Be honest with yourself. The results and benefits of the practice are not in the future in an image of what and how you think you should be practicing. It's happening now;
- See the correlation with how you move and relate to your body on the mat and how you move and relate to your body in life, off the mat. Write a few words;
- Observe whether you hold onto postures even though it does not feel right. If so, why?
- Can you feel the difference between healthy yoga challenge and an egoist approach? What is it? How can you move beyond these limiting habits, if they occur for you?;
- Are you able to find your individual fit through personal reflection or do you always look for the guidance of the teacher?;
- Are you able to cultivate and nourish an attitude of benevolence and respect for your body in balance with challenging yourself and moving beyond beliefs that keep you stuck?; and
- With all of these inquiries can you see a correlation with how you practice and how you live your life? Write a few words. Date your entries.

Look at your practice from these different perspectives:

1. Focus on the heart centre, on compassion and practising as devotion. See how this manifests in all your postures, and write about it. Notice how your heart centre feels in different postures, such as when you are able to release or when you hold back. Can you practise with love? Why?
2. How do stability and strength manifest in different postures? Do you feel stable on your mat? Do you feel stable if you fall out of a balancing posture? What determines your centre of stability? Write about the difference between strength and rigidity;

3. Reflect on flexibility. How do you determine whether you feel flexible or stiff? Can you feel the importance of being flexible in balance with strength, without favoring one? Do you see a connection between your mental flexibility, and your physical flexibility? Do you consider yourself flexible? How flexible do you want to be? Where is the source of this flexibility? How can you feel its fullness? Right now do you feel stable and flexible?;

4. Be present to your body temperature. Some postures are cooling, some our warming. Can you tell the difference? Do you crave warm or cool air? Would you say you have more internal heat or that you have more of its opposite? Do you feel in balance?; and

5. Inversions enable you to see things from a different angle, and experience your body upside down. What are you focusing on when you are inverted? Do you have the ability to take on different perspectives in your life off the mat? How does that serve you? Do you see a correlation?

Always return to these questions. Answer them honestly, let them go. Look at another aspect and then return to the beginning. See if anything has changed and write about it.

We are also taught to focus on the *manipura chakra*. To understand this let us look at the word *cakra*. Adapted as chakra for the English language *cakra* has a few meanings. In this case, it denotes vortexes of energy associated with different centers of the body. In Hindu-based yoga texts, seven chakras are emphasized. They are:

1. *Sahasrara-cakra* (thousand-spoke wheel) located above the crown of the head;

2. *Ajna-cakra* (command wheel) in the centre of the head between and behind the eyebrows;

3. *Vishudha-cakra* (pure wheel) at the throat centre.

4. *Anahata-cakra* (wheel of the unstruck sound) at the heart centre;

5. *Manipura-cakra* (wheel of the jewel city) at the navel centre;

6. *Svadhishthana-cakra* (wheel of the self base) at the genitals; and

7. *Muladhara-cakra* (root-foundation wheel) at the anus.

Each of these psychoenergetic wheels relates to our subtle experiences, and we can bring balance and vitality to them through awareness, mantra practices, meditation, and yoga asanas. Creating an association, a distinct state of consciousness, which brings life to the experience, is essential. Practise the chakra cleansing meditation as taught in class daily, and write about your experiences (speak with a knowledgeable teacher if you have not taken the course).

As for the subtle aspect of the *chakras* look at your life through the following lens:

1. *Sahasrara-cakra* (divinity, God, and beyond concept): Do I relate? How does this impact me?

2. *Ajna-cakra* (intuition): Do I trust mine? Do I know its voice? How does this impact me?

3. *Vishudha-cakra:* How much willpower do I have? Do I have confidence in my word? How does this impact me?

4. *Anahata-cakra:* (benevolence, compassion, and love): How do I give and receive them? Am I open to love? How does this impact me?

5. *Manipura-cakra:* How much confidence do I have in myself? How does this impact me?

6. *Svadhishthana-cakra:* Am I comfortable with my sexuality? Do I express my creativity? How does this impact me?; and

7. *Muladhara-cakra:* Do I feel safe and secure? Do I trust life? Am I comfortable in my skin? Do I feel connected with nature? How does all this impact me?

The practice of hatha yoga also asks us to see, and remember divinity, to be humble and devotional.

For Reflection

What is your relationship with devotion itself? Do you feel devoted? If so, what and or whom are you devoted to? If not, why not? Do you want to express devotion? How can devotion be expressed consciously and daily? How about devotion to life itself as an appreciation for the manifestation of all life? Can you see the beauty, the perfection, and interconnectedness in all life? What types of daily practices could you implement to bring this practice to life? How can you breathe life into your everyday living? Devotion requires very few words. You could pray to remind yourself, but really devotion is an attitude that underlies our every action. Can you see it? How does it manifest for you?

Attitude

*If, in the presence of circumstances that are about to
take place, you can take the highest attitude possible
— that is, if you put your consciousness in contact
with the highest consciousness within reach, you can
be absolutely sure that in that case it is the best that
can happen to you. But as soon as you fall from this
consciousness into a lower state, then it is evidently
not the best that can happen, for the simple reason
that you are not in your very best consciousness. I even
go so far as to affirm that in the zone of immediate
influence of each one, the right attitude has power to
turn every circumstance itself.*

The Mother

Chapter 5

The Four Golden Sisters

Concentration, Patience, Silence and Discipline

Concentration

The ability to zone the mind on one thing, and keep it there is not only one of the most powerful practices we can nurture to succeed on our path, but it's an essential component. Think about it, how far can you get if you have no ability to see what, and where you really want to go? Concentration is calm, active, energizing, free of tension, and is a catalyst for meditation. To experience true concentration it must be practised, and the recognition that we can always improve allows us to dive deeper into the experience. It's easy to see that without concentration it's very difficult to achieve anything. Here is a simple example to see concentration in our daily lives: Imagine that you are at a busy, and noisy restaurant with someone you find fabulous. Chances are you would not be distracted by the activities and sounds around you. You would instead joyfully keep your focus, your attention on her. On the other hand, if you were at that same restaurant with someone you have little in common with, you may find your mind wandering looking for something more interesting to fix itself on. Like a puppy, what is that smell? Who is over there? Continuously stimulated and unable to focus.

As mentioned, I began journaling as a teenager, using my journal to write affirmations. I believe in affirmations, but without adequate concentration, without inner cleansing, and questioning these affirmations had little impact on me beyond making me aware of what I was craving, and that what I was craving was often based on what I thought was the secret to a happy life. Learning to concentrate, to go within and sustain the focus made me realize that a lot of the things I thought I wanted, I really did not. Concentration cleanses our psyche, but understand that it must be practised to bear fruit.

In addition to the importance of paying attention to what matters, Patanjali tells us that concentration is one of the antidotes for the mentioned obstacles. Patanjali explains that we can concentrate on gross objects, subtle objects, bliss or I-ness, but that in essence the single point of concentration is your choice, but again, commitment is essential to reap the benefits.

The following point of focus is offered by Patanjali: concentration on the universal sound of om. Om is a composite of the letters A+U+M; its recitation is one of the oldest and most practiced yogic techniques. To practise, know that when you repeat the sound of "A", which is "A" as in "father (not "A" as in "and") you focus your energy at the heart centre. When chanting U (as ou) the focus is at the throat and the vibration of M is at the head. The M is long and meaningful, similar to the natural "mmm" sound that comes from eating a ripe fruit. There is also a moment of awareness on the silence as the M comes to an end. At this point, the focus expands out to the crown of the head.

If you are new to this practice, repeat this mantra out loud. If you do not enjoy the sound of your voice, whisper. Once you have some experience you may be able to practice in silence and still focus. Alternating between out loud, whisper, and silent is also a good practice.

An example of such a practice is: two minutes out loud, two minutes whisper, three minutes silence, two minutes whisper, and two minutes outloud. The inconvenience with this method is that it requires an awareness of time. I prefer to trust my inner clock, but you can choose to use a timer. Alternatively, you may simply practise outloud, whisper or in silence. Only with repetition and practise will the method bear fruit. Merely reading and knowing of the method will not!

Another benefit of concentration is that it helps shift draining and limiting thought patterns. It's not uncommon to believe and to teach that positive thinking is about turning a negative belief into a positive one. For example, one could easily believe that the technique to transform hate is to reverse it to its opposite, love, as we often think of love as the opposite of hate. However, we must understand that love never hates. Love is pure. The opposite of hate is "non hate", and if we approach trying to "non hate" when we are having such an intense feeling, we may be able to fool ourself, but chances are we will be trying to cultivate an opposite mental energy using the same aspect of the mind. Cultivating the opposite means redirecting the energy within as opposed to using the same external search engine to try and create an opposing feeling. This must be approached with patience, calmness, focus and discipline to bear fruit.

For example, you are in a situation where you feel very angry at someone and you are having negative thoughts towards that person. Changing the thought patterns to visualize yourself forgiving this person and filling her with love and light is one method, but better yet, move away from the fragmentation of the busy mind and go within to your centre. With regular practise concentration on one single point will create the opposite feeling as opposed to using the same distracted fragmented mind to create concepts and try and convince yourself that you have created a change. You may, on a certain level, but it may be more of a translation than a transformation. Which means you may simply be using different words to express the same feeling as oppose to creating a true shift. Be honest with yourself.

For Reflection

Think of things in your life that draw your attention and be aware of what you focus on. Do you concentrate on wants and needs or gratitude and respect? What draws your attention, love, fear, faith, or worries? Ask yourself what thoughts, sounds, images come up when you try to concentrate? Could those be harnessed or channeled? For example, if you notice song lyrics in your head, could you use mantra to place meditative sounds at the fore before trying to meditate or concentrate?

Patience

To concentrate we need to cultivate patience. Patience is a synonym to wisdom. Wisdom is defined as a deep intuitive understanding of life and our relationships that is beyond conceptual knowledge. Patience is a catalyst and a result of grace, effort, intelligence and understanding. I was speaking with someone who was expressing extreme impatience. As a joke she says: "When God was passing out patience I was behind the door and he missed me." It's not uncommon to make light of our imperfections, but in this case, a statement like this gives us the permission to continue and entertain this belief system, therefore, sets our limitations.

Patience is a virtue worth cultivating. We don't need to be religious to see and experience the power of time. None of us are immune to it. Our material world is constantly being eaten by time. Time as we know it has the benefit of creating order in our society, but true time is relative and changing. Patience opens our eyes to this illusion and provides us with an inner experience of letting go of our expectations and reminds us to keep up regardless of time expectations.

Here is an example of how I cultivate patience: I love my computer, but fixing computer issues is not something I enjoy. Even when it comes to adding software I would rather let someone else do it. Because I value patience and want to nurture it, I try as often as possible to move beyond this. To take my time, read the directions, breathe and patiently add or remove what needs to be done. Provide examples for yourself and put them in action. Then return to the journal and write about your experiences.

For Reflection

How would you rate your starting point with patience? Are there situations where you are very patient and others where you find it more challenging? For example, some people have incredible patience when it comes to fixing, building, creating, etc., but when it comes to people, not so much. For others, it's the opposite. They have a tremendous amount of patience for people, but quickly get irritated with little things. What about you? How and where can you cultivate this virtue?

Ask yourself what regularly tries your patience? Is this a clue that something has got to give? Are you building in enough self care, or could you better address your needs to be able to move forward and practice patience? Are there any other obstacles to patience? What would taking on a practice of patience look like for you?

Silence

The practice of silence is called *mauna* in Sanskrit. It's an external practice that eventually becomes an internal experience. Until that inner silence is achieved, the attitude underlying the silence determines the experience. We have all seen and experienced the effects of negative silence, including: awkward silence, silence meant to withhold information, arrogant silence, or the type of silence that ripples out from low self esteem. The silence recommended for this practice is heart centered, kind, and compassionate. It's the type of silence that supports the experience of inner silence.

As we become aware of the amount of energy that is expanded through our thoughts, words, speech, and tone of voice we choose wisely how to manage and nurture our energy. So much of our vitality is expressed through our communication and having moments of silence brings this to life. There is a reason the word noise comes from the Latin *nausea*, meaning seasickness.

We are creatures of habit and easily become accustomed to the everyday noise that surrounds us. Sometimes we may even feel we have stopped hearing it. However, every sound and every word impacts our energy. As we create more and more moments of comfortable silence we feel how very true this is. We notice the impact that our words have on our body and relationships. We start to choose with care what we will contribute and know when silence is best. I encourage you to give yourself the gift of silence everyday. No one is too busy, I assure you. It's possible to make it fit. Be creative. Start small and see it unfold because silence is profound and may be one of the reasons we often choose to avoid it.

For Reflection

Be aware of the sounds you consider interesting and invigorating and the sounds that drain your energy. Be aware of the sounds you have control over and the ones you do not. Are you comfortable in silence? Do you look for external stimulation? Look at times and places in your life where you could enjoy some silence and instead choose sound. Are you open to giving this practice some space in your life? Why? It takes patience to move beyond the initial discomforts and intensity of silence, but the benefits far outweigh the initial challenge.

Ask yourself, when do I naturally find silence? How could I introduce more silence into my life at my home and at work? How about taking care not to over schedule yourself, or taking a silent walk at lunch rather than seeking company? How about turning off the television, and radio just to eat in silence when you are home alone? Also remember to worship your words and use them wisely. See the impact they have on you and those you share time with. Open your ears to the beauty of silence, and write some thoughts about your experiences.

Discipline

I recently spent some time with someone, who has next-to-no discipline. Due to this lack of discipline his finances, health, and relationships are all in a shamble. Yet, if he sees something that is well packaged, and attractive he buys it, continuously spending on trinkets. He eats what he chooses, never reflecting on the value of what he is eating, the impact that his food choices have on his well being or on our environment. Everything is in the moment, there is no patience for anything, he is simply always looking to please his senses.

I mentally compared his lifestyle with that of someone else I know who is quite disciplined, wondering how can one person be so disciplined, and another have so little discipline? This inspired me to bring up the subject of discipline and the value it has on our life. He had never reflected on discipline and asked if I thought that the lack of discipline was negative. He could not understand why I value discipline and thought of it as a negative word, associated with guilt and being reprimanded.

Spiritually speaking, discipline sets the path and prepares us for our growth. Some claim that enlightenment can be spontaneous and that any effort towards 'it' is a distraction. How can that be? If we look around us, very few people spontaneously experience inner bliss.

What do we have to gain from discipline? If we make efforts to move beyond simple sense gratification, we start to see how easily we can be influenced. Through discipline, we train our minds to concentrate and go within, and see what we surround ourselves with. Know that keeping a journal is a discipline because it requires an honest, and regular investment on your part, and to take what you reflect on, and integrate it in your everyday life brings discipline to life. Always remember that discipline is not a dry, and rigid practice. It's a balanced energy of effort and letting go, of mental strength, and flexibility supported by benevolence.

For Reflection

How do you define discipline? Do you consider yourself a disciplined person? How is it manifested? How could you improve? Do you want to improve? Discipline takes effort, and to get a sense of the amount of effort it takes try applying the following:

Rise 30 minutes earlier than you normally do (unless of course you are already an early bird. I do not want you rising at 3:30 a.m.). There is nothing like creating that shift to show us the amount of energy that is required to move forward. Rise, and greet the day. Take deep breaths, journal, meditate, go for a walk and/or enjoy nature. Whatever you choose, simply wake earlier and be in silence – no radio, television, or children – just you and silence. Write a few words about your experiences.

Another way to feel the depth of discipline is to avoid gossiping and complaining. Upon rising make that commitment, saying out loud in a convincing, and honest voice something like, "Just for today, my words will be kind, truthful, and of service. I will abstain from gossip and complaints." This may sound easy, but you will quickly see how much energy we waste on poor speech and how easily we sway to unnecessary and mindless chatter. This effort will also allow you to feel the depth of discipline and like a muscle, the more we work it, the stronger it becomes. Write a few words about your experience.

Chapter 6

The Gunas

My intention is to provide you with a short, and yet, concise and clear understanding of the *gunas*, allowing you to use the wisdom for personal introspection. The word *guna* has many uses, but in this case it's translated as qualities of nature. There are three qualities to nature: *rajas* (the energy of action); *tamas* (the quality of inactivity and inertia); and *sattva* (the quality of purity). These three qualities are present in nature as a whole, including our food, our body, mind, emotions, life itself, and so forth. In short, they manifest in our body and mind as such:

An unbalanced *rajasic* person is ostentatious, indulgent, enjoys rough, and demanding exercise. The mind is restless, agitated, self asserting, disputatious, and on the emotional level quick to anger, ambitious, overly assertive, and prideful.

A *tamasic* body has a sloppy appearance, lacks in exercise, and can even be unclean. On the mental level one is dull, ignorant, and likes to unnecessarily argue about petty things. Emotionally, *tamas* brings about fear, paranoia, depression, and hatred.

A *sattvic* body is flexible, vital, strong, pure, and benefits from gentle exercise. A *sattvic* state of mind is demonstrated through mental clarity, a perceptive nature, an ability to focus and remain honest. Emotionally, *sattva* is loving, faithful, generous, compassionate, and loyal.

Rajas is more positive than *tamas*, but not as positive as *sattva*. These three qualities exist in all beings and are a part of nature's manifestation. Everything has a beginning, a middle, and an end. There exists an energy that brings these qualities to life (*rajas*), a sustained and exalted beauty (*sattva*), and a closure or death (*tamas*). The degree and combinations in which these qualities manifest continuously vary.

As taught in the *Bhagavad-Gita*, when *rajas* is dominant we are full of cravings, and attachments. When *tamas* is dominating heedlessness, indolence, and excessive need to sleep arise. *Sattva*, on the other hand, is happiness.

However, know that a *sattvic* state is not the goal, but it's the tool that allows us to start integrating the deeper aspects of yoga. One of the benefits of self observation, study, healthy nutrition, yoga asana, and meditation is that we awaken and sustain for longer periods a *sattvic* state. As this *sattvic* state awakens in us, we have more physical energy, more mental clarity, more patience and understanding. Forgiveness is easily expressed, and it's natural to go within. The interest in this journal is a sign of *sattva*. *Sattva* is part of nature; breaking down and rebuilding, but the more *sattvic* a lifestyle we live the more we see this cycle manifest in ourselves and our life and this quality of observation nourishes *sattva*.

"Arise, awake, and stop not 'til the goal is reached!" is one of the central teachings of *Vedanta*. To awaken we must first rise. Nothing will change through *tamas*. It takes *rajas* to create a shift. Too much *rajas* creates imbalances and destruction. It's a fine balance. Look at yourself, and your life with honesty, and benevolence. A good place to begin and see these energies is to look at your diet. As mentioned, food either has a dominance of *tamas*, *rajas*, or *sattva*. As we eat, food becomes a part of us, and creates that energy through us. Typically after a Thanksgiving meal you feel heavy, tired, and sluggish; the result of eating too much, and of eating heavy food that is devitalized and "dead" and thus creating a *tamasic* feeling. Think of how you feel after too much caffeine – a nervous energy pulsating through your veins - supporting the depleting side of *rajas*. Because we are creatures of habit, we may think that these sensations are normal and some may even have forgotten what balanced energy feels like, and find themselves going from one extreme to the other. Without a set point, we may not know what we are missing.

For Reflection

Take some time to become aware of your dietary choices, and how they impact you. Write from an energetic perspective. For example, for breakfast I had this, and within this time I felt that. Did you feel energized, content, heavy, anxious? In a way it's simple, if a food is dead such as refined flour, dairy, overcooked vegetables, or heavy oils it makes us feel lethargic. You may be full after such a meal, but you are rarely satisfied. If it's a stimulant such as sugar, caffeine, or additives you may feel stimulated, but inevitably you will crash.

With *sattvic* food, there is no crash or lack of balance. If a food is fresh and full of nutrients when you eat it you feel alive and satisfied. A *sattvic* diet is nourishing; it includes fresh fruits, vegetables, whole grains, legumes, and adequate hydration. Sitting calmly when you eat you take the time to chew, eating until you feel content and satisfied. Recognizing that if you do not eat enough, you will feel tired and possibly irritated and if you eat too much the same occurs. Wanting food to be nourishment, providing sustained energy and vitality you take full responsibility for your choices. Also, the cultivation of a *sattvic* attitude is essential. There is no sense in cultivating an attitude of guilt and expectations towards wholesome food.

See these same energies manifesting in you. When we are *sattvic*, we feel energized, awake, clear, and able to relax fully. When *rajas* dominates aggression, frustration, destructive, and negative competitive thoughts and actions lead the way. Relaxing becomes very challenging, therefore, the experience is more of a collapsing nature. Living like this encourages the potential for burnouts. When *tamas* dominates depressions sets in. We feel heavy, tired, and discouraged. It's very difficult to move beyond *tamas* once it has set in. See it in yourself and promise to rise, to wake up, and keep up. Life is so short, why not try?

If we don't take care of our body, it has a tendency to become heavy, and tired (*tamasic*). If we don't take care of our mind, it is often unable to focus, always searching, and looking externally for some form of distraction (*rajasic*). It's possible to have a *sattvic* mind, and a *tamasic* body. Look at yourself and find your balance. Going back to my undisciplined acquaintance (mentioned in chapter 5), I also noticed that he was sighing and exhaling loudly with every action. Everything was an effort. Whether it was getting in the car or getting out of the car, serving himself a coffee, or trying to figure out what to watch on television, everything was an effort. He had no interest in learning anything new, not even learning how to use the remote control for the television. I saw firsthand how heavy *tamas* can be, and it's not attractive. Honestly, I was at times disgusted, and this made me look at myself even further.

My disgusting meditation
"I was sitting in meditation clearly not meditating. Instead, I was thinking about my undisciplined friend, justifying the negative thoughts I had towards his lifestyle. I was convincing myself that I was not being judgmental or cruel. I was simply being honest and sometimes honesty hurts. In my head, it made absolute sense. At one point, I could see the thought process as opposed to being taken by it, and I then decided to observe the impact that it was having on me physically. This is what I noticed: My jaw and my posture were tight. My shoulders were rolled forward, and I felt "dirty". I would love to provide you with a better example, but dirty was how I felt. I thought, "I wonder what he is seeing in me?" What kind of projection am I providing? I then started to think where I was at 15 years past. I thought of the teachers that inspired me, and none of them made me feel disgusting. I know that I would not have benefited from such a behavior. Then I thought of some teachers that are having an impact on me today and realized that they never look at me with disgust. Subsequently, the thought, "who do I think I am?" instantly softened my edge. I spent a few minutes in meditation bathing him with *prana*. I made a promise to myself to repeat a mantra whenever I noticed my mind going on its tangent or whenever I felt the desire to express my frustrations out loud. I also noticed that to let it go I had to feel it fully. I had to ask myself who is feeling disgusted? Where is this coming from? Through this questioning much was understood."

It also led to the following reflections that I encourage you to reflect on.

For Reflection
How often do I sigh? How often do I choose not to learn something new out of laziness? How do I use my body? How often do I feel heavy, and that daily tasks are a burden? How does all this impact my relationship to my life?

I had a friend who was always looking forward to vacation, working for the possibility of vacation and never really enjoying work itself. Another form of *tamas*.

Look at your day: how many of us rise feeling tired and heavy (*tamasic*), fill the body with caffeine (*rajas*), work neurotically with the feeling that if we are not manic, or in a panic, we are not being productive and then go home and crash, collapse, and associate this collapsing with relaxing? It's not only possible to be productive, and mentally calm, and clear, but it's our true nature.

To evaluate what kind of energy sustains you, answer the following questions:

For Reflection

Are you able to relax? Are you always tired? Do you care about yourself and life? Are you overly competitive? Do you sleep well? Do you sleep too much? Do you awaken feeling refreshed and alive? See it in yourself. How do you feel about yourself right now? Are you worried or content? What is your body language saying? Open your eyes to the play of the *gunas*, and let your intuitive knowledge lead you. Write about this cycle and how you see it manifest in you and your life. How does *sattva* feel? How can you nourish a *sattvic* state? Remember no attachments or expectations!

> *"The body has a remarkable capacity of adaptation and endurance. It is fit to do so many more things than one can usually imagine. If instead of the ignorant, and despotic masters that govern it, it is ruled by the central truth of the being, one will be surprised at what it is capable of doing."*
> The Mother

Chapter 7

Ah...The Mind

To deepen our understanding of our self we will look at the different aspects of the mind referred to as *manas, citta, ahamkara,* and *buddhi.*

1. **Manas:** Relates to the activity of the mind that regulates, or supervises the senses. It's not meant to direct, therefore, it's always looking for direction, and will listen to the loudest and authoritative aspect of the mind;

2. **Citta:** The aspect of the mind that collects information, and stores it away as memories. When this aspect of the mind is not in balance with the whole of the mind, its countless impressions float around drawing attention, and create all sorts of wants and needs for *manas* to carry out. Often, these desires are only habitual and they are rarely useful;

3. **Ahamkara:** This aspect defines itself as separate. Known as the small ego it creates partnerships and separations based on the information stored in *citta*. This mixture can create all sorts of fears and painful experiences. *Manas* often finds itself carrying out the desires stored in *ahamkara*, which are made up of feelings of individuality leading to separation and supporting competition and comparative behaviors. It's known as "I-am-ness"; and

4. **Buddhi:** Is our deepest wisdom and intuitive knowledge. Always knowing when to discern, when to judge and the direction to take leads us on a journey of inner peace, and contentment. The challenge is that it's often clouded by the loudness and activities of *ahamkara* and *chitta*. Keeping a journal helps to hear its voice and know how to trust and follow through on its wisdom.

To bring deeper meaning and understanding to this information, practice the following guidelines:

For Reflection

1. Manas: Be mindful of your actions and speech. Notice how your senses (smell, sight, touch, hearing, and taste) lead your actions. Most of us have a dominance in terms of the sense we tend to use to experience the world. A good way to know which sense leads your day is to write a couple of paragraphs about your day. Write what you did and how it unfolded. Then look for key words. Do you express yourself through feelings? For example, I awoke energetic, looking forward to my day as I knew I would accomplish my goals. Alternatively, when I woke up

this morning it was still dark. I took some time to look through my notes to help me remember where I needed to be. Do you recall the visual, or are you kinesthetic? How do you communicate to the world? What is your language? How does your language impact your actions? Again, know what draws your attention and recognize that with mindfulness you can focus on what matters.

2. Citta: Pay attention to the waves of your thoughts to connect with *citta*. Notice how your thoughts come in and return to where they began. Notice the thoughts *manas* relates to and the ones that are like clouds moving along without any attachment. We have thousands of thoughts moving through our mind, most are repetitions with little value. But many come in and attach themselves to an emotion, love or its opposite, and once this happens it impacts our energy as a whole by creating a belief. It becomes part of what we identify with, therefore, dictates our journey. Write a few words (11 words or so) about your childhood. Do not think about it too much, avoid judging it. Just see what arises. Then see if there is a correlation with these words and the way you relate to your everyday life. Keep writing! And remember always date your entries.

3. Ahamkara: Our thoughts are often colored with either an attraction or an aversion. I like this but not that. I like her, but her? No! I am this, and capable of this, but that, no, and I can't do that! Be aware of what you like and do not like and whom you like and do not like. Write it out. Write out 11 attractions and 11 aversions. See if you can uncover their roots. Where did these associations stem from? How are they serving you? Do you see any association with your 11 words of childhood?

4. Buddhi: You will see buddhi begin to shine its lights when bondage begins to reduce. Eventually, bondage fades away fully, and we are no longer attached to the results of our actions. Thoughts of separation fade away leaving us with the experience of mental clarity. Although the experience of unity is beyond mental chatter, write some thoughts regarding unity and mental clarity. Do you live intuitively? Can you hear your inner voice of wisdom? Do you feel calm and clear? When? How does it manifest?

We can see that if we approach life with *ahamkara* or *citta* guiding *manas*, desires meant to support our ego lead our actions, even when it comes to keeping a journal. This is why it's so valuable to understand how our mind works, and see where our intentions are coming from. If I journal from an egocentric place of desires meant to support my neurosis, then of what value is journaling? Now ask yourself who is this "I" that wants to journal? Where is this desire coming from? What do I hope to gain? Can I release my attachments?

The more you work with this and see your mind at play the more you will be aware of the five *vrittis* of the mind (sutra 1.6). *Vritti* can be translated as circular patterns of consciousness. These patterns are: correct knowledge based on sound reasoning; misconception (e.g., we see a shadow ahead believing it to be a person, but as we approach it we see that it is a bush); imagination; memory; and deep sleep. All of these can be experienced with or without pain. For example, recalling a painful experience versus recalling a happy memory. As you pay attention, you will quickly see how true this is. Watch your mind, where is it, ahead or behind? What types of memory do you focus on when you recall your day? Do you focus on what serves you or what limits you? Regarding imagination, what do you fantasize about? How does it serve you?

"A strong conviction is necessary that `I am the Self,
transcending the mind and the phenomena."
Sri Ramana Maharshi

Chapter 8

Equanimity

These days, balance has become a common term to evaluate our life. We seek it out, and feel in or out of balance based on subjective perceptions of what we have conceptualized as being balance. For example, it's not uncommon to equate balance with having our family life, work, rest, exercise, etc. in perfect harmony, feeling that this is the achievement of successful balance. As we all know, moments of external perfection based on expectations are fleeting, and this quest for the impossible combined with the absence of reflecting on what balance really is creates a distorted search that leaves us feeling unsettled.

Sutra 1.12 is the foundational practice to everything we approach. Basically, we are asked to: always keep up and yet always let go in balance.

In Sanskrit, the word for practice is *abhyasa*. *Abhyasa* is about always keeping up with our practice regardless of thought processes that may want to keep us away. Maintaining good intentions is something to cultivate and nourish in your everyday life. Recognizing that every activity we engage in requires energy is the beginning of creating balanced energy. Some activities take a tremendous amount of energy and give us very little in return. Examples include such things as worrying, complaining or gossiping. These activities require energy, take energy away from our centre of balance, and then create a downward spiralling energy. We practise instead silence, uplifting communication and gratitude. We begin to experience more inner peace, and are then able to keep up with our practice of eventually stilling or observing the fluctuations of the mind. This is very empowering because we experience our true nature beyond mental agitation. Set an internal environment for practice, remember that when we begin something new, we need to invest more energy to develop the habit. Once we have it, the memory faculty reminds us to practice listening to *buddhi*. In short, the essence of *abhyasa* is the practice of cultivating that which brings us to the experience of mental stability.

To help with the process write what thoughts, words, and actions lead you in the direction of mental stability. For example, rising feeling nervous, agitated, and anxious about what needs to be done, choose to have a coffee and read the paper. Or rising feeling nervous, agitated, and anxious about what needs to be done, seeing the mental pattern for what it is and choosing to take a moment of silence and stillness, breathing, connecting with nature or meditating and journaling. Then, having a coffee and so on. Choose thoughts and actions that will help you keep up, even when the mind pulls you away. What will it take for you?

For Reflection

Write what thoughts, words, and actions support mental instability. For example, "I don't have time for this. It's too painful to sit here and breathe and feel the anxiety in my core." What types of thoughts will stop you? Now that you can see it clearly make a commitment to yourself to choose what serves you.

To reap the benefits from our steadfast effort (*abhyasa*) it must be in perfect balance with non-attachment. Always keep up, and always let go! Renunciation is the practice of non-attachment from desires (sutra 1.15). In Sanskrit, the word for non-attachment is *vairagya*. In doing this work, most of us have a desire to attain something. Whether it be inner peace, happiness, or enlightenment, but something is drawing us. This is of service as it has taken you here, but you must let it go. Any attachment to expected results will keep you distracted and looking for a concept you have created about what you think you want. When we let go we are able to move beyond these expectations and we start to integrate the essence of our steadfast effort with more ease.

For most of us, letting go is not easy. Beginning with external factors to see the process unravel helps to cultivate the habit. As a mother, I see this with my daughter in balancing the amount of dedication to her, the ability to let go, let her have her experiences, and make her own choices. When we cultivate this balance externally with concrete aspects of our life, we have a sense of what it means with our inner journey ("As within so without and as without so within."). Be present, love, let go, and trust. I remember one year setting the intention to have the courage to give, and receive love fully. When I thought of that intention, it felt great. I started to journal to help me get a sense of what that would be like. I quickly realized that this was the only way to love. Either you love or you do not. Really think about it, how could one not love fully? It makes no sense. Love is perfectly balanced.

It's good to understand the difference between non-attachment and indifference as it's easy without adequate reflection to confuse them. Remember that non-attachment is supported by practice. To see these two qualities blending together (as opposed to two separate entities) helps us grasp what is being taught.

For Reflection

Write your definition of non-attachment. Write your definition of indifference.

Non-attachment happens in stages, or in cycles, it's an unfolding process. For example, I had a friend who used to get very upset when she would let someone pass when driving and they would not express gratitude. Being able to let someone go without expecting anything in return is a simple example, but a great place to start.

Look for places in your life where you could let go of expectations. Write them out.

Start small to build a good foundation and then let it grow from there. Just as when we want to strengthen our biceps, we begin with lighter weights and as the muscles strengthen we increase the load and are able to maintain good posture, energy and proper breathing. If we were to begin with too much weight, the foundation would go, and we would give up or get injured.

Let go. Say it out loud: "I am willing to let go, and I trust in the process of life." Say it again. Feel it in your heart. As you start to cultivate it externally you will begin to see clearly what you are attached to, and how your attachments impact your decisions, and your overall energy and personality and the awareness brings forth freedom from the attachment.

The more we balance practice, and non-attachment the more space we give to *buddhi*. When this aspect of the mind leads our life, we begin to receive the gifts of yoga. These gifts include a variety of *siddhis* (siddhi is an unusual skill, faculty, or capability). One of these *siddhis* is *uha sidhi*, meaning clear thinking and correct understanding. This is worth the effort. Think of all the time we waste due to poor communication, even with ourselves.

We can then feel that true balance is the radical acceptance that the only certainty in our everyday life is uncertainty. When we have a direct experience with being in balance, we realize that it's as much about appreciating the smooth times as it is about remaining centered in chaos and accepting that this also shall pass. The experience of balance is directly interconnected with contentment, happiness, and peace, which are all beyond the pleasing of the senses.

To tap into the experience of balance, we need to take responsibility for our individual choices, and free ourselves from the limiting thought patterns that often govern our decision making. Acknowledging that life is fast, the media is loud, and our economy is often driven by excessive mindless consumerism keeps us awake to what is happening around us. Who wants to wake up one day to realize that s/he is a slave to the things that were created to serve her/him? I doubt life is about continuously trying to fill a void to experience fleeting pleasures that may leave us feeling full at times, but never really satisfied.

This popular anecdote was created to emphasize the point that we look externally for what can only be found internally: "There is a man bending down on his front lawn looking for something. He seems quite desperate. His neighbor walks by and asks if she can help him find what he has lost. Graciously accepting he says, "I have lost my keys and have been looking for quite some time". After a few minutes of patient searching, the neighbor asks if he is certain he has lost them out on the front lawn. This is when he lets her know that he has actually lost the keys in the house. Baffled, she now wants to know why they are outside looking for them. He replies, "It's dark inside I can't see a thing."

The following is a short and true story: My husband and I were sitting on a patio at a coffee shop talking with some acquaintances. All of a sudden, the young girl at the next table started yelling, and frantically running around the patio. She had spotted a bee, and was clearly agitated. As she ran and yelled, her dad remained seated with his head down, looking embarrassed by the situation. The small dog at the next table then started to bark and run around, obviously troubled by the situation. The young girl then jumped into her father's arms for respite. The woman (our acquaintance) at the next table then jumped up and started accusing the owner of the dog for barking at the young girl, and possibly biting the girl (the girl had no marks and had said nothing about this potential bite). The owner of the dog then started yelling profanities at the woman. You can see where this is going. An entire chain of reaction based on fear.

For Reflection

How often do similar situations happen in your everyday life? How frequently do you react, when you could have responded? What if the above mentioned felt in balance and knew how to respond to life? What do you think would have happened? Write some thoughts about reacting to life and responding to life. What is the difference? What do you see in yourself?

There is no doubt that all feelings are part of the human experience. It's what we do with the feeling itself that determines whether the experience will be of service, or a detriment to us. For example, anger can be used in negative ways towards ourselves, towards others, or it can be a tool of inspiration to create valid shifts.

> *Even a knowledgeable man acts according to his own*
> *nature; all living entities are controlled by their own*
> *nature. What can repression accomplish?*
> Bhagavad-Gita 3.33-

Take the time and contemplate this. What can repression accomplish?

The good news, as you know, is that we have the ability to create shifts through mindfulness, and observation. In Sanskrit, the word for mindfulness is *smriti*, and it also means memory. Therefore, to be mindful we must continuously remind ourselves. However, it takes work, and a willingness to shift and grow.

Another important ingredient for integration is relaxation. I must say that I had no idea how much I needed to relax until I started to let go. We have all read the articles and seen the statistics regarding the impact negative stress has on our life. We know it, and yet it's so easy to be looped in, to be swept away by its energy, and in the process lose our sense of inner balance. Relaxation is essential because as we let go of tension we naturally return to equilibrium. When we feel centered and calm, our productivity increases, our mental clarity improves, our creativity shines through and all of this ripples out and impacts the people we love.

For Reflection

Define relaxation. What do you currently 'do' for relaxation? Write about the correlation between relaxation, peace, and contentment. What does a relaxed you look like? Can you be at peace and productive? According to Yogis, real peace is always unshakable. What do you think of this?

Define stress. What do you do for stress? How do you cultivate it? This is not a mistaken question. We need to be aware that we not only create stressful situation in our life but we support them. Possibly feeding them through our belief systems, and our actions, continuously repeating past patterns. Therefore, write out what you do to nurture the habits? How does stress feel? What stresses you the most? What can you do about it? Do you see a positive side of stress? Do you see how it could be of service to you?

Do you believe that you have what it takes to be a clear, calm, focused, energetic, and peaceful person? Why? Where does your belief come from? Describe a peaceful environment. Describe a stressful environment. Have you ever felt stressed in a peaceful environment? Have you ever felt at peace in a stressful environment? Can you clearly see how what we focus on grows? Without a doubt, our external environment impacts our inner vibration, but our inner vibration has a bigger impact on our experience. Awareness is key.

For example, I know that when my mind wraps itself around something to worry about it does not matter much where I am because I am in my head inventing things around my issue to worry about. I compare it to my dog getting a scent of something. Taken by the smell, I call him, and it takes a moment for him to snap out of it. I do the same thing. I grab a hold of what is worrying me, and just get right into it, oblivious of my surroundings and use my worries as a meditation. I am happy to say that I can often see myself being taken by it, and feel how my entire energy changes, and through this observation I have more ease with letting it go. The more I meditate and journal the faster I catch myself. However, don't take my word for it, explore for yourself.

I remember going through a minor health issue, using Google as a source to try, and help me figure out what may have caused my discomfort. One of the underlying causes was stress. My first thought when I read it was: "That does not apply to me. I am not feeling stressed." At that moment I noticed that my teeth were clenched. Good thing stress was not an issue! Something tells me I am not unique.

Commit to the experience of daily physical relaxation. It can be as simple as taking the first 10 minutes when lying in bed at night to guide yourself through a relaxation. There are so many methods and possibilities that can be integrated in any busy schedule. The most important piece is that it actually be practised. As you start to feel your body release tension that you may not have been aware you were carrying, you will inevitably start to feel lighter, and mentally clearer. This will then ripple out with increased energy and patience resulting in making fewer mistakes and craving fewer caffeinated drinks or sugary treats. Thus reducing the demands on the liver and adrenals, consequently increasing your overall energy. You see the spiral effect it creates?

For Reflection

Write out your daily practice to relax your physical body. Take your time. Know yourself. What will you actually practice? Be true to you. Write in your journal what your daily relaxation practice will be and commit to it.

As time passes review your written commitment. Did you maintain it? What was the result? What did you learn? What challenges or obstacles arose? Were you able to identify them and move beyond them? What have you released? Date your entry and review it frequently.

> *"Yoga teaches us to cure what need not be endured and endure what cannot be cured."*
> B.K.S. Iyengar

Chapter 9

Investment

I t's not uncommon when we begin something to be tempted by future results, which means we end up being more interested in what we think we are going to gain rather than what we are actually engaged in. This tendency can easily lead us on a draining, and distracting path. The awareness that our starting point is the tool that took us to the practice, but that it does not need to be our main motivation, is what will support further integration of the practice. When we began our yoga practice, or any other spiritual journey, something had to draw us to it, and that something was a reflection of our starting point. For example, today we see ads with pictures of beautiful people practising yoga, or meditation all dressed in white on a sandy beach. The ad reads something like "inner peace is for you". And we think, I want that! I want beauty, and inner peace, and so we sign up for a class or a retreat. If we do make it to the beach retreat, we quickly realize that internally our mind is still the same. We may physically be at the beach, but mentally the vibration that we entertain is still there, pulling. We soon recognize that this will require some work on our part. Signing up and showing up are an important and essential beginning but it quickly becomes obvious that to tap into this inner peace, we will need to invest more energy, and unconsciously we then choose how much we are willing to invest in our practice. One thing I have learned along the way is that my willingness to be disciplined is what risks a plateau not the gifts of the practice.

The following is a common, and true example. A new student to yoga comes into the centre. She is a high-strung 55 year old. With intensity in her eyes and voice, she tells me her doctor recommended yoga because she has high blood pressure, and she needs to learn how to relax. I reassure her that she is at the right place. She commits to a class pass, coming once a week for about four weeks. Then it's about twice a month because she is very busy. After about four months of practice she tells me that she does not think that yoga is working because her blood pressure is still high. I sit her down, clearly explaining that she needs to come to class at least three times per week, and that she also needs to integrate some of the teachings into her daily life.

I explain that yoga is a lifestyle practice and that if she is willing to invest some of her energy, stress management is just the beginning of yoga's gifts. She agreed and today is a transformed woman. Not only is her blood pressure down, but her eyes are softer, her breathing is deeper, she is kinder to her staff and family, and has begun a meditation practice. She needed to know that it would take more investment on her part.

As she experienced, the return was worth it! We all need to accept this and take the leap. Show some commitment and discipline. See the circle of our life. See how one thing impacts the other and so forth. Be present and take responsibility for your actions.

Also, take the time to reflect whether you really want what you are striving for. For example, On occasion when people ask I provide "email yoga life consultations." I am sharing this most recent interaction with you, with *anonymous* permission. I am paraphrasing, but I am keeping the essence of the revelation.

I was asked: "I don't understand why I still suffer from anxiety and lack of sleep when I have been practicing yoga for almost 12 years. Why am I not receiving the full benefits?"

After a few emails, we quickly realized that my anonymous student 'sorta' believes a regular yoga practice can bring her to inner peace, and she gives 70 percent when it comes to regular practice and commitment and she does not really understand "inner peace." A part of her sees it as a "boring" state that older people access, and she likes being fun, youthful and active.

Therefore, it became very clear through introspection that she is wondering why she is not achieving a goal she does not really want through a practice she sorta believes can take her there while investing only 70 percent of her energy!

For Reflection

What about you, do you know what you want? Is there a possibility that you already have it? Is there a possibility that you don't really want what you 'think' you are after? How much energy are you willing to invest? Really take some time and think it through. Write about your energy levels and what you are willing to give up and what you are willing to improve upon. How much energy will it take to make the change? Do you have extra energy for it? Where will it come from?

As we know, simple things such as rising 30 minutes earlier, taking some time to meditate, and/or journal is quite energizing, and yet how often do we choose to sleep in? We all know that if we eat well and avoid evening snaking that we will sleep better, rising with more energy, and yet how easy is it to indulge in that evening piece of chocolate, or glass of wine? Really take some time to look at this. This practice is not about guilt or restrictions to create alienation, and lack. It's about true happiness and returning to our centre of balance in a world where we so easily get pulled in unnecessary, and limiting directions.

Remember that introspection is like cleaning your house – the more you get into it, the more conscious you become of the dusty corners. However, just like making an effort, and cleaning your home well is rewarding, so too is taking the time to explore your habits. And like cleaning your home, even if you spend many hours and fully dedicate yourself to create an immaculate home, it will not last. You will need to continuously repeat the process. However, as we know, regular maintenance makes it more manageable. Again, concentration, silence, patience and kindness mixed in with the reminder that life is short keeps us focused.

At this point in your journey, I encourage you to take a pause and kindly remind you that this is not a race, and you will not be done once the journal is complete. Be patient and take your time. Get to know you and how you relate to your world. Review what you have written and start over. See if anything has changed.

For Reflection

Reflect on the value of investment. Reflect on what, and where you currently invest your energy. What kind of return are you getting? I have a friend who thinks I am foolish for choosing not to financially invest in corporations I find immoral as they are the ones providing the best return. What she does not realize is that the value on the return is based on what we individually value.

Ask yourself what is important to you. Look at your daily life, and be conscious of what you invest in. This includes simple everyday activities you entertain such as conversations, nutrition, rest, exercise, and friendships. How many of your regular chosen activities bring you a healthy return? Do you feel inspired by your friendships? Do you feel energized and loved by your family? Remember this is about you, what you put out and what you allow in.

"To listen to some devout people, one would imagine that God never laughs."
Sri Aurobindo

Chapter 10

Morality

Not a black and white subject, but an essential component of personal exploration. It's easy to see that our moral and ethical values guide us through our day and these values shape the decisions we make inevitably impacting our actions. These daily actions have a ripple effect and create a karmic imprint that further determines our perceptions of what we experience. The following is a list of a few of the moral fundamentals of Patanjali's wisdom, which are recognized by most schools of yoga. I include some of my thoughts and reflections only to spark your thoughts, but essentially this is your book. What is important is to know what and why you believe what you believe about the following points and be aware of the ripple effect your beliefs have on you and your life as a whole.

Ahimsa (nonviolence): Although nonviolence is mentioned in the earlier *Vedas*, it was not until Patanjali included it as the very first aspect of the very first limb of his eight-limb path that we see a developed philosophical account of nonviolence. We translate it as nonviolence, but most scholars, philosophers, and masters of yoga agree that it means so much more than our understanding of nonviolence. It's also important to understand that this was a guideline for already very advanced students. Therefore, our understanding and ability to implement nonviolence is one that is continuously unfolding as we ourselves grow and expand our awareness of ourselves and this world.

If I ask you whether you consider yourself a violent person, chances are your opinion will be based on comparison. It could be the world at large as seen through the eyes of the media. It could be by comparing yourself to a group of people or one person. The questions you must ask yourself are how high is my bar, and who am I using as a role model? Also, it's very easy to find news about violent actions taking place throughout the world, and it's possible that our fear of being victims to it creates a form of anxiety, which then impacts our daily patterns.

A Documentary

I was watching a documentary about one of the most dangerous gangs in the prison systems. They were interviewing one of its original leaders who is now in a segregated part of the prison system for his protection. This man has been incarcerated since the age of 20. At the time of the interview he was in his 50s. He will be in prison until his death. Prison life is what he knows. He has brutally killed numerous people and was the leader for many murders outside the prison walls even while in prison. At one point, he turned against his gang, which is why he was now in protective custody and has been there for the last 15 years. This is what he had to say, "I have nothing against violence when it is among people who understand and live for violence, but I will not support violence against innocent people." You see his gang had decided that they were not only going to order murders on other gang members, but that they would also have wives and children of their enemies be tortured and killed when necessary. He felt they went too far. He had found his limit and was now living in fear of being killed by what he created.

Living nonviolently requires reflection and it requires faith. I believe that when we act with violence, we are often reacting out of fear, therefore, a lack of faith. Whether my violence is manifested as negative thoughts towards myself, as a total disregard for Mother Nature, or whether it's pure violent actions towards another human being, I believe it stems from some form of fear. This is why in my reflections on nonviolence I always ask myself what is it that I fear?

We all react differently, some people express their aggression with obvious actions, while for others it's more subtle (it is what we call passive-aggressive behavior). I strongly believe that we all have the dignity to live peacefully. This means it begins with our thoughts, which then ripples out to our speech, and then to our actions. It applies towards I, you, and it. Yogis teach that as a we become firmly grounded in nonviolence, other people who come near us will naturally lose any feelings of hostility.

I know from experience that we must have a definition of nonviolence that requires regular review. The more peaceful we become, the more aware we become, and our definition evolves with us. Blind spots become more and more visible with time.

For Reflection

Define nonviolence. Do you consider yourself a peaceful, caring, and compassionate person? Who are you comparing yourself to (are you comparing yourself to the status quo)? Are you willing to aim higher than what is considered to be socially acceptable? What if we, as a nation, were to raise the bar? What would that raised bar look like? Do you believe in our human potential for pure nonviolence? Where does your belief stem from (i.e., personal experiences, books, articles, the news)? How do think your belief is impacting you on a day-to-day basis?

When you listen to your thoughts are they of a peaceful nature when you think of yourself? Look at your family life, how is peace being upheld at home? Is it possible to find peaceful and uplifting confrontation and is it a choice? What do you think about our potential to live peacefully? How does your belief impact you and your life? What you think matters because this is what leads you.

I have observed in myself that one of my traits is to avoid confrontation (not for nonviolence issues, but simply because I have issues with confrontation) at all cost, and I end up suppressing energy and it ends up building resentment, which then ripples out in detrimental ways. Whether it be physical pain, fatigue, depression, or sarcasm towards those I love it does come out. We all need to remember that nonviolence does not mean being a passive doormat. Kindness towards yourself and having the courage to be true to yourself can be challenging. To try and move beyond this, I have been nurturing my ability for on-the-spot forgiveness. It's a great feeling. Instead of making believe that I am okay with a situation when I am clearly not, and instead of simply putting it away in the heart vault, I forgive right there and then. It's of course easier with small things, but it does feed the habit.

For Reflection

Do you believe that we are peaceful by nature and somehow forget? What would a pure nonviolent you look like (think of your eyes, your smile, and your posture)? Are you willing to improve? If yes, how much energy will you need to invest for your improvement?

Where will this energy come from? If not, why not? What's important is to set attainable goals, and watch yourself meet these goals. Be present to the impact you have on people; before speaking take a breath. Ask yourself, is this an improvement on silence? Is this worth the energy?

Vegetarianism is the recommended yogic diet. I have read that it's human nature to try to have the best result with the least amount of energy exerted. Well then, according to many researchers, such as the largest study ever conducted on human health and nutrition The China Study by Dr. T. Collin Campbell, vegetarianism fits in with this model. Not only is it a healthy and clean diet, but it's a sustainable diet that requires less energy from Mother Nature. Plus, we have seen what the over-consumption of animal protein is doing to the animal kingdom. Therefore, by opting for a vegetarian diet we: bring healing and nourishment to our body; honor the animal kingdom; respect Mother Nature; and by reducing our needs we have an impact on reducing world hunger.

For Reflection

One simple thing, but so much in return. What do you think? Do you agree? Why? There are other such examples of how we can have very positive impacts with little effort. Look for them. Create a list for yourself.

Satya (truth): This *sutra* tells us that if we always speak the truth our words will always bear truth. It's quite something to be honest, fully honest. To be fully honest, we need to be aware of the lies we tell. Have you ever listed the number of times you lie in a day? This includes silent lies, little white lies, exaggerations, and outright lies. One of the ways I work on improving and speaking my truth is by paying attention to my speech. I notice how I feel after a lie, reflecting on how this lie served me and who I lied to. I ask myself what I was trying to protect or gain by lying.

Then I practise telling the truth when it would have felt so sweet to share a lie. I look at my posture, notice my voice to gain an understanding of my habits and of my fears. A lie can be taken so far that the entire image is a lie, having an idea of who we think we should be and putting on a mask to face the day. Being who we think people want us to be. There is a saying that goes: "worst than telling a lie is trying to live up to a lie".

I have a friend who cannot stand social media for this reason. She cannot move beyond the masks, the portrayals that people create about themselves, showing just what they want you to see. Of course, there are many positive aspects of social media, and not all is persona, but she does have a point. Plus, we see images in the media, and may feel that we do not compare. We need to open our eyes and see the difference between persona and authenticity.

Is honesty a quality you seek in a person? There is a business owner whom I visit, who is creative and devoted to her work, and I just love talking with her when I am in her store. She is also a pathological liar. My daughter asked me once why I choose to talk with a liar. I told her that she has many other qualities, and we all have imbalances. When the business owner starts her story telling I simply choose not to entertain the subject, and I kindly bring it back to the moment. I also reminded my daughter that people don't always lie to manipulate or be harmful, some lie out of personal protection or out of a belief that the truth is simply not good enough.

For Reflection

Are you honest? Ask when you choose to lie what is it that you are trying to protect, or gain. Do you have a persona? What would be the benefit of such a thing? Do you view having a persona as a positive attribute? Do you have the courage to be you fully? Can you connect with, and accept the perfection of your individuality as an interconnected source? Where do lies begin and end? What is the value of honesty? How do you feel when you speak the truth when you were somehow convinced that a lie would have really improved the story? What is your current starting point? Be honest now – this is just for you. How can you improve? Give yourself a goal. The mind likes goals because it likes to know where it's going. Provide some direction for yourself.

I was looking through my closet, not finding what I wanted. I said out loud, " Time to reorganize." Although I often hear Swami Sivananda's wisdom in my mind, "Never put off to tomorrow what can be done today." I said out loud, "Tomorrow is the day." The next day at 9 p.m., remembering, and realizing that I had not reorganized, I got up and did it. I want to use my words wisely, and have faith in what I say. Even when it does not seem so important.

Asteya (non-stealing): We all know that stealing is inappropriate. Most of us would not steal a car, a bank or someone's jewelry. But, how about, you are at a coffee shop owned by a very rich corporation, and the barista gives you back too much change? Do you keep the extra change? What if this coffee shop was a small business, would you keep the change? Does the size of the business make a difference to you?

There is also theft of words and knowledge, such as taking someone's knowledge, and claiming it as our own. Stealing ideas, copying without asking, or acknowledging are all forms of theft. Withholding information that would be of value to someone else is also a form of theft. For example, during some of our *satsangs* (uplifting gatherings), some employees of large corporations shared that withholding information is normal behavior, and really the only way to get ahead. Questions to ask are: get ahead of what?; and what kind of normality do we want to be a part of?

When we let fear lead the way, we can lose ourselves. The mind's limitation creates an "us", and "them", therefore, a form of violence.

For Reflection

What do you think? Look in the mirror, picture yourself at five years old. What would you tell yourself? Now picture yourself 20 years older, what would your senior self say?

Here is an interesting dilemma for morality: About 20 years ago, a friend had just been accepted as a military police, undergoing intense training. During training, he was asked the following question: "Your father has lost everything, the world is struggling, and you catch your father stealing a loaf of bread to feed himself, and your mother. What do you do?" The answer they were looking for was: "You turn him in." I asked him if he would. Without hesitation, in a very stern voice, he said yes. This is why I remember our conversation.

Here is another example to reflect upon: Over the years as a yoga centre owner, I have met thousands of people. I can remember two lovely people who did not like spending money. These two students came to class twice weekly for years. They always expressed so much appreciation for the classes, and my knowledge, but when it came time to renew their class passes, that was another story. They never had their wallets with them.

They would always (always is not an exaggeration) forget to bring their wallets to renew for at least two, or three weeks. When they did remember there was a lot of sighing and negative comments about money while signing the cheque, and they both always asked for a discount. To forget once is acceptable since we all forget. Forgetting twice works out as well, but every time, for years? My friend claimed that it was my energy that was allowing this behavior to happen. Two people out of so many? I am willing to own up to my limitations, but some people are attached to their money to the point that it can become a form of theft.

For Reflection

What do you think? Do you look for deals at the expense of others respect and dedication to providing services? Where is your line? Regarding Mother Nature, what is your relationship to her? Do you ever steal of her bounty out of laziness, or greed? Do you think you have enough? Have you ever been a victim of theft? If so, how did it feel? List examples of when you have stolen, and how you felt? Now set intentions for healthy and trustworthy habits.

Aparigraha (greedlessness): Non-grasping is taking only what you need and being willing to let it go. When we first reflect on non-grasping or greedlessness we may think of material possessions, reflecting on the relationship we have with them, and our possible desire to accumulate them.

For example, I know a few people who own enough pairs of shoes that they lose count of what they have. However, they find themselves entertaining and identifying with this shoe fetish with so much pride and pleasure. When I listen to them speak, I often think that they are more attached to the story and their identity as "shoe people" than they are to the actual shoes. Therefore, one could argue that they are not only clinging to the shoes themselves, but that they are clinging to the identity of being shoe fanatics. You see, non-grasping means non-grasping in every way.

For Reflection

Most of us cling onto people, material things, and our perceived identity. What and whom do you cling to? See yourself. Ask yourself what ideas or belief systems you are clinging to. How are they serving you? What is it that you need? These are big questions. Try and visualize yourself using only what you need and trusting in the process of life. See yourself letting go of people and allowing them to be free of your expectations. Try and think beyond social conditioning. Think about it globally, what if we all agreed to simplify? Can you picture it?

While out on a walk my daughter expressed gratitude, and respect towards having such a strong and supportive family presence in her life. I knew that in my situation I did not have to be her everything. Any mother knows how challenging it can be to let go and trust because the instinct is to protect, and nurture our way. Yoga taught me to let go. It taught me to love fully and let others do the same, to never give up, and always let go. We were both blessed with loving people around us. I chose to let it flow; she noticed and felt grateful. Every situation is different, but within these differences we can find our place, our centre of gravity. These examples are only meant to show balance within variety. What is valuable is for you to look at your life, and find areas where you may benefit from letting go.

I have come to believe that much of the suffering we see is based on greed – the greedy and poor suffer because of it. Letting go and non-grasping are certainly worth your time to reflect upon. We start to experience that the more we let go the more we unite. Again, I must remind us all that the more we reflect, and the more we put this into practice, the more we actually understand the depth of it. However, we can only start where we are. One step at a time while moving forward.

Tapas (heat or glow): Historically, when a reference was made regarding a yogi, it referred to an ascetic or a *tapasvin*, describing someone who practiced strict penance rather than a philosophical orientation towards enlightenment. The word *tapasvin* comes from *tapas*. *Tapas* can further be defined as the endurance of extremes, which is why we may see, or hear of extreme feats. However, in the yoga *sutras* and the *Bhagavad-Gita*, *tapas* is positive, and does not create, or support destructive practices. *Tapas* is healthy, self discipline, and purification and it's fair to say that *tapas* is anything that moves us beyond robotic sense gratification.

To improve we must contemplate our current lifestyle and see where we could benefit from cleansing. The daughter of a friend had chronic asthma to the point that she had to be hospitalized a few times. They had her on all sorts of medication trying to help, but it was not until they moved that she uncovered mold in her daughter's bedroom. The asthma pump was never needed in her new home. I know that as I purify my environment, I am inspired to purify my body and mind, and the cycle is manifested in all directions.

Again, I see in myself that there are layers of purity. Without the full experience of purity, our understanding of purity has a shadow; without acknowledging the shadow we may become attached to our current understanding, and prevent further growth. There are so many ways that we allow impurities in our life. For example, I have seen some movies I wished I had not seen simply because of the memory imprinting.

For Reflection

Take some time to define and write about environmental physical and mental purity. Remember, thinking and writing are two different things; we see so much more when we write. Your home, car, office, body, and mind are not garbage cans. How can you keep them clean? Diet, exercise, breathing techniques, conversations, material you choose to fill your mind (media, books, and movies) are good places to begin exploring. What can you let go of in your home? It took me years to be able to keep organized files. My starting point left me feeling cluttered and utterly intimidated at the thought of organizing them. Where can you begin the cleansing process both internally and externally? Write out what you will commit to, date it, review it, and continue to add. Is your house perfectly clean superficially? What if we open a drawer? Are there similarities with how you feel?

You may not relate to the examples I am giving, but I am trying to start a pattern of observation for personal questioning. Based on your starting point, state one thing you are willing to improve upon. Once you are satisfied with your progress, add another. See the ripple effect that it has on you. Write about the ripple effect.

The Sanskrit term for a householder is *grihastha*; it's a term developed as a promise to the aspirant that yoga is not only for those who retire to the cave and as mentioned, both *Patanjali* and the *Bhagavad-Gita* regard *tapas* as a positive practice. They do not endorse extremes or practices that create imbalances in the body, which can be the case in extreme asceticism.

The *Bhagavad-Gita* states that *tapas* of the highest order include offering service to God, and your spiritual teacher, purity, honesty, continence, and nonviolence. Those are the disciplines of the body. To offer soothing words, to speak truly, kindly, and helpfully, and to study the scriptures are the disciplines of speech. Calmness, gentleness, silence, self restraint, and purity are the disciplines of the mind. When these three disciplines are practiced without attachments to the results, with dedication, and faith, they are *sattvic*. When disciplines are practiced to gain power or respect, or when they torture the body, they are either *tamasic* or *rajasic*.

Finding balance with our *tapas* takes reflection. I had the privilege of receiving initiations from highly established yoga teachers. During one of the breaks at a level one training in *kriya* yoga, the teacher told the class that he believes in the middle path. In his 40 years of practice, study, and travel, he has met people who practice extremes and found many imbalances and much unhappiness. That is something many accomplished yogis seem to agree upon.

For many of us, the practice of the middle path is quite attractive. I see it as modest, honest, and most importantly, accessible. However, in its quest it's essential to be aware of the aspect of the mind that has an innate ability to justify anything, and to find loopholes simply to win the case and support the senses. The awareness that if we want something badly enough, or if we have a limiting belief that is ingrained, the desire, the habit can easily be supported and justified is what allows us to move beyond it.

This is why it's vital to have reflective time. The acknowledgment that what we deem as the middle path is highly determined by our starting point keeps us honest. Now let us look at the how of asceticism for the householder. We will look at the body, the mind, and our lifestyle by exploring *tapas* as self discipline, and purification. We know that purification is required at the level of the body and the mind. It's an easy self-test. If our body is sick, heavy, bloated, anxious, and so forth, it takes up a lot of our energy leaving one with very little energy for other endeavors. If the mind is filled with complaints, worries, and greed, sitting still and reflecting can be painful.

On my journey, I do my best to live in balance, nurturing self discipline to support my mind and body. When it comes to purifying my body, I have experienced extremes, and in retrospect see that it turned into a neurotic obsession, even toxic on a mental level. I had a student who believed in the power of nutrition to the point that her entire health relied on it. She ate a perfectly clean diet, never ate anything that was remotely "impure". Her diet allowed her to maintain a very low body weight and she had beautiful skin, which made her feel successful. However, she continuously complained, had a tremendous amount of resentment, and had all sorts of physical pains. You see, she did not take care of her mind, only her body through extreme nutritional belief systems of guilt and comparisons. Some things come easily for us, but unfortunately may become imbalances if taken too far. Balance, introspection, silence, and honesty are essential. It's also beneficial when we start cleansing the body, to be clear on our intentions. We must be honest or we may give up or move to extremes, which are equally detrimental.

Let us compare our body with our home. Imagine that you went to visit a friend at her home. Upon arriving, she showed you her front porch with great passion and knowledge, telling you everything about the details, the workmanship, the flowers, and the type of paint. When you requested to see the backyard she asked you to climb on a ladder and get a peek of it through a hole in the fence. When you asked to see inside she replied, "We can't go in there. I have no idea how to turn the lights on.", I think you would find that strange. But, that is often the relationship we have with our body. The relationship is one dimensional (such as the front porch). We only focus on the back if it hurts. And, in relation to the inside, well, we leave that to the experts.

Let us go back to our imaginary friend. What if she also had a love for garage sales, buying up all sorts of junk, opening the front door to her house and stuffing it in there? Eventually, some odd smells and noises might come out from the house. In response, our friend simply buys more aromatic flowers, incense, and plays louder music to mask the smells and noises. I am sure you see where I am going with this. We cannot continue to fill our body with excess junk, and simply wear perfume to mask its odor. We really must get acquainted with our body as a whole, and treat it as a home we can never sell, until of course "the day".

I know from experience that the practices of self discipline and purification are an unfolding process. For example, there was a period in my life when it took tremendous self discipline to stop smoking and eat more green vegetables. Today, I have created the habits, experienced the benefits, and feel well established as a nonsmoking, green veggie lover. Now I have time and energy to look at other aspects of my physical health.

An accessible cleansing method is diet and nutrition. Simply not overeating provides great respite for the body. Eating whole foods instead of processed foods along with a vegetarian diet is considered optimal. It's important to look at your starting point and the relationship you have with food. Keeping a food diary for a week or two sheds light on your habitual patterns. Once you know your starting point the purification plan can begin. It just takes a little self discipline.

As the *Bhagavad-Gita* tells us, yoga is impossible for him who eats too much, nor for him who does not eat at all, nor for him who sleeps too much, for him who is always awake. Yoga becomes the destroyer of pain for him who is moderate in eating and recreation, who is moderate in exertion and actions, who is moderate in sleep, and wakefulness.

For Reflection

What do you think of moderation? Do you agree? Do you consider yourself moderate? Why? What do you base this on?

The practice of asana (yogic postures) is also recommended. Our bodies are designed to move. Bodies are not created to sit 14 hours per day. There is an intelligence to our body, and its mechanics that yoga asanas honor in a way that no other physical practice does. There are many excellent teachers; it's all about finding the style and teacher that is right for you. Stay grounded and flexible, and begin or continue the process attentively, and with kindness. Question your starting point, set goals, and stay committed.

As for the mind, there is no doubt that it will benefit from the efforts placed on cleansing the body. As long, of course, as these efforts are done with care and respect. But also the mind needs special care.

Remember *Sutra* 1.6 tells us that the movements of the mind are fivefold: valid knowledge; inverted knowledge; imagination; memory; and sleep. The experience of these can be painful or non-painful. For this purpose, let us emphasize the memory and imagination aspects of our mind. We are highly influenced by our environment and our social conditioning. The memories we choose to hold onto, and entertain are in many cases based on these elements. These elements highly determine the experience of our current conditions.

When my daughter was young I played mantras with the intention of filling her mind. She was raised vegetarian since birth. I have always been very honest with her as to why I chose this diet. This way of eating was not very popular 18 years ago and some worried that I was brainwashing her. My answer was always the same – we are all on some level brainwashed. We seem to think that if it's a collective agreement, then it is the way it should be, and we often associate this collective agreement with free will. However, if it's different then we may choose to view things as radical. There are many examples of socially acceptable choices that are not acceptable, but we choose to accept these choices without question simply because there is a majority of acceptance.

Many of our belief systems are based on an unreliable faulty memory, and then we use our imagination and create all sorts of stories to support our belief systems. The stories are often based on these false memories that were highly influenced by other people's experience of life. Like anything, memory can be of service, or it can be a detriment, and the same goes with our imagination. This is why it's essential to acknowledge that today's experience becomes tomorrow's memory. Let us try and pay attention to what really matters. Let us try to express gratitude, be kind, smile and forgive.

We too often simply accept our beliefs as our truth, believing everything we think. Unfortunately, our culture values the accumulation of knowledge and facts at the expense of intuitive living. It's obvious that some knowledge is worth collecting, but a lot of it is useless, meant only to titillate perpetuating mindless sense gratification and consumerism. What do you think, do your experiences determine your beliefs, or do your beliefs determine your experiences?

For Reflection

To help purify the mind ask yourself, how do I start my day? What do I focus on upon rising? To help further our questioning, let us read the passage on tapas from the *Bhagavad-Gita* again. *Tapas* of the highest order include offering service to God, and to your spiritual teacher, purity, honesty, continence, and nonviolence. Those are the disciplines of the body. To offer soothing words, to speak truly, kindly and helpfully, and to study the scriptures are the disciplines of speech. Calmness, gentleness, silence, self restraint, and purity are the disciplines of the mind. When these three disciplines are practiced without attachment to the results, and with dedication and faith, they are *sattvic*. When disciplines are practiced to gain power or respect, or when they torture the body, they are either *tamasic* or *rajasic*.

Here we have it, *tapas* at its best. Let us look at this with deeper personal reflection. Soothing words, being kind and helpful. Do you see yourself as someone who provides such support for yourself and others? Write about the difference between kindness and niceness. In my opinion, there is a big difference between the two qualities; I aspire for kindness. What do you think?

Continence can be defined as moderation. Again I ask you, are you moderate? I love cycling, and sometimes I cycle quite a bit. I notice that my energy changes because the more I cycle, the more aware I need to be about what I eat, and when I eat it. I eat more and need more rest. Cycling too much impacts my body with some neck stiffness, which at times impacts my sleep. Therefore, it impacts my life as a whole. Although I love being on my bike, I feel much better overall when I keep my cycling in balance. Moderation, give it some thought.

What about gentleness? I was at the grocery store, and the cashier, unaware of his brisk movements, was grabbing my food, and almost throwing it on the other side as he was scanning it. How do you move? If we think of how much we use our hands on a daily basis, and ask what do I touch, grab, or feel? Recognize the amount of energy that resides in your hands. Think of how good a loving hug feels. How do you share your gentleness with yourself and others? What about practising with dedication and faith? How does that look like for you?

What about your home environment? There is a popular saying that goes, "We have become slaves to the things we have created to serve us." Our possessions can own us in many different ways. Firstly, the clutter it creates in our home becomes a reflection of the clutter in our mind. Secondly, the amount of work required to maintain it drains our energy and our resources. Thirdly, the self identification with possessions tends to keep us from identifying with our true nature. Lastly, none of these possessions brings full satisfaction, and yet we tend to keep looking outside ourselves, believing and hoping that the next acquisition will somehow fill that void.

I have accumulated many books over the years. I felt attached to them all, never complaining about moving them. A time arrived when due to plans for an extended period of traveling, I really had to reduce my collection of treasured books substantially. I went through the collection carefully, clearing out about 30 books, feeling as though that was enough of a purge. I thought the remaining books were essential to my life. However, I realized that this was not a possibility, and got rid of another 40. Again, the pattern repeated itself, and I got rid of even more. Now, although I had a sense of attachment to these books, I can hardly remember the ones I gave away. As well, I have rekindled my relationship with our local library. What a wonderful service. The reminder that a householder's asceticism includes the reduction of materialistic accumulation reminds us to pay attention before making our next purchase.

I know two people who are both financially very prosperous, and have the freedom to purchase (almost) anything they want. Today, they find themselves owning homes, cottages, cars, motorcycles, sporting equipment, and businesses that are all falling apart. They have so many material possessions, but no time to care for them. Unfortunately, that also includes their family, friends, and work relationships. I am not saying that all wealthy people find themselves in this situation. Still, their example is not unique. Of course, some people have very little wealth and still find themselves in a similar situation. Our current social acceptance encourages this way of life. If we do not take a look at ourselves from time to time, if we do not take a moment to examine how we are treating the things, and most importantly, the people in our lives, we easily can end up in similar situations.

For Reflection

Do you own your possessions, or do they own you? How many possessions do you have that you really need? You can start the clearing process with anything such as books, clothes, knickknacks, or sports equipment. Once you start the process it becomes easier; you then question before making a purchase. Start in one room. Look in the cupboards you are unable to reach and see what is up there, Do you have anything that has not been of service to you in a long time that could be of great service to someone else? Believe me, purging is liberating. It impacts our whole life when we live in a home that is clean and clear. Also, see the union between your body and mind. How does this union manifest? Where is the mind located?

Samtosha (contentment): When I started my yoga practice, and would encounter contentment in the writings, I would skip the chapter. If the topic arose at a training

I was attending then I would go to the washroom, or daydream. I did not want to hear about contentment. I believed that if I was content, I would stop growing, stop striving, stop being fully human, and fully alive.

Eventually, I started to experience a level of acceptance, of contentment, as a ripple effect of my practice of asana, meditation, *etc.* It was a liberating experience; not only was I still showing up for life with commitment and dedication, but that I was actually more present. What I experienced was that through contentment, I was more open. The fear of failing was not as much of a motivator, which brought some mental freedom for the beauty and perfection of what was. This direct experience created a genuine interest in contentment, and I learned that contentment means being in balance between hardship and ease, it has nothing to do with giving up. That is quite something.

The more contentment we experience the less demanding, or needy we are. We see the beauty in our current experiences and stop looking beyond them at what we think we should be having or doing. It's amazing what we can miss when we leave the room, or skip a chapter simply because we have already created our own definition.

For Reflection

Take some time to define contentment. Say out loud right now, "I (insert full name) am content." How did that feel? Are you convincing? Did your tone of voice and posture support your statement? This time, repeat it as you look in the mirror, in your eyes. Again, how did that feel? Simply reading this and imagining yourself saying it out loud will not do. Listen to your voice.

I believe that contentment is freedom. Contentment right here, right now, exactly the way things are. What do you think? Is it a possibility for you?

This poem is inscribed on the wall of Mother Teresa's children's home in Calcutta, India. The poem is attributed to her, however, it is believed that the original version was written by Kent M Keith.

People are often unreasonable, illogical and self-centered;
Forgive them anyway.
If you are kind, people may accuse you of selfish, ulterior motives;
Be kind anyway.
If you are successful, you will win some false friends and some true enemies;
Succeed anyway.
If you are honest and frank, people may cheat you;
Be honest and frank anyway.
What you spend years building, someone could destroy overnight;
Build anyway.
If you find serenity and happiness, they may be jealous;
Be happy anyway.

The good you do today; people will often forget tomorrow;
Do good anyway.
Give the world the best you have, and it may never be enough;
Give the world the best you've got anyway.
You see, in the final analysis; it is between you and your God;
It was never between you and them anyway.

Because our culture highly values productivity, we may feel that if we are content, we will stop producing, therefore, stop being part of society. This is a misunderstanding. Through reflection, observation, and the willingness to see the extraordinary in the ordinary we can move beyond this mental belief and give ourselves the space to experience our true nature. If you sit for a while and contemplate the opposite of contentment what arises? What does lack of contentment do for you? Is it of any service besides possibly being habitual? Mother Teresa is quoted as saying," Be faithful in small things because it is in them that your strength lies."

Ishvara-Pranidhana (surrender to God, sutra 2.45):

When we moved to our new home I felt overwhelmed by what needed to be done. I was happy to be with my husband knowing that he felt calm and had clarity in terms of how it would unfold. When we look at a project from every angle possible, it's easy to get discouraged, to feel that the task at hand is just too big.

Be aware of the big picture, but also be aware of your potential, and integrate it calmly and creatively knowing that you are moving forward even when you may feel that you have come to a halt. Think of all the things that are repetitions in your life (e.g., eating, sleeping, hydrating, etc.) which regardless of how well you perform them, will continue to require repetition. For example, we can't stop drinking water because we have been drinking it for the last (x) number of years and give up because we don't seem to be soaking it up. We know that it comes in, nourishes, and flows out. So does our inner work; it's not a temporary journey promising an eternity of wisdom. It's a daily task, and like breathing, and hydrating, we can neglect it, and then wonder why we are so tired and irritable. It's a choice.

I have experienced feelings of inadequacy as I approached my journey, and I know I am not alone with this. Remembering that practise itself is heartfelt, therefore, perfect allows me to move beyond these limiting beliefs. We do not need to be anyone else, or experience anything else, other than what we are.

For Reflection

How does living devoted to God sit with you? Do you have a relationship to this? Why? What does this relationship or non relationship look like for you? How does it manifest in your day-to-day activities? Do you believe in this? Why? Where did your belief stem from? How is it serving you?

Being able to understand the written teachings is called *adhyana siddhi*. *Adhyaya* means to study, furthermore, it is intuitive understanding, right understanding, and knowing what is hidden in the written word to complete the meaning. Again, we see the importance of cleansing and clearing to have a new beginning. This work will help clarify and remove some of the blinders that may prevent you from either wanting to study and meditate, or will deepen your current experience and understanding of your study.

Another essential component in this section is what Patanjali calls *Swadhyaya*; study of the self. This journal is a practice of self study and asking: who is studying? Who is reflecting? What do I want? And why? As well as, asking who am I and answering *neti neti* (not thus not thus) to everything that arises will help further your practice.

> *"The highest stage in moral culture at which we can arrive is when we recognize that we ought to control our thoughts."*
> Charles Darwin

Chapter 11

The Four Aims of Life

With an understanding of ourselves and a sound moral foundation, we are ready to look at the four *purushartha* (four aims of life). *Purusha* can be translated as the unchanging aspect of who you are. In the *Shambala Encyclopedia of Yoga*, Georg Feuerstein states that the *Gopatha Brahmana* defines the word *purusha* as "he who rests in the castle". The castle being the body. The following definitions for the four *purusharthas* are defined in *Mantra Yoga* and *Primal Sound* by David Frawley:

1. **Dharma**: One's primary purpose, vocation, work, or career in life;

2. **Artha**: Achievement of necessary goals and objects, including wealth, property, to facilitate one's dharma;

3. **Kama**: Achievement of happiness and fulfillment of desires, including relationships, family, and children that support, express, and expand one's *dharma*; and

4. **Moksha**: Liberation of the spirit, and self realization, which is the highest goal achieved mainly through the practice of yoga, meditation, and the fulfillment of our *dharma* as an immortal soul.

We will now review each of the *purusharthas* for the moral householder.

Dharma

To discuss dharma we need to ask the question that is on everyone's mind, what is the purpose of life? One of my favorite answers (given by a variety of spiritual teachers) to this question is: The purpose of life is to live your purpose, and your purpose is individual. Therefore, we can say that on a certain level, each and everyone's purpose is unique **but that living with purpose is the true purpose of life**. On a deeper level, we accept that our collective purpose is freedom from the limiting thought constructs that keep us stuck and separate. However, the path we take, the life we live, is 100 percent unique. How freeing is that? It's such a wonderful way to approach life because it removes the urge or habit to compare ourselves to others and allows us to be our own self. As mentioned, we waste energy and stray from our individual path when we continuously look outside our self to try and connect with life's purpose, my life, my purpose.

Remember that purpose does not necessarily equal recognition. This is a likely confusion. The desire to be recognized by others can lead us to feel inadequate even when we are living our truth. Patience, commitment, and an open mind and heart provide wise guidance. Trying to skip growth stages, moving too fast, creates resentment and instability. Accepting phases of life and opportunities nurtures true balance.

As the quote by Howard Thurman (philosopher, author, and theologian) reminds us, "Don't ask yourself what the world needs, ask yourself what makes you feel alive because what the world needs are people who feel alive." Living with awareness connects each of us with our sense of purpose; thus, feeling balance from the inside out.

Life flows and realizing that having choice means an abundant lifestyle opens our heart. Accepting that the expression of our *dharma* evolves, as we and the people we serve evolve, grow, and live. Expressing gratitude for the gifts we do have and looking at the beauty of our experiences brings inner peace and supports healthy choices.

A few years ago a student asked for a private class to reflect on life. She explained how unhappy she was at work and how frustrated she felt about life in general. After some discussion, it was obvious that the profession she was in did not happen by accident; she worked hard to be where she was. I asked her if all of her decisions had been made through fear. She assured me that they had not. We started a list of what she loved about her work and soon concluded that there were many things she wanted and appreciated from her profession. What she resented the most was the lack of creative opportunities. I asked her if her profession ever promised creativity; she smiled and said no. Realizing that this was equivalent to being upset because her cat did not bark she felt a sense of ease instantly. Financial security and stability were very important to her; she loved routine and felt respected at work. The uncertainty of an artist's life is not something she would be willing to experience; thus, she now allows for artistic creativity in her personal life and feels more balance. We all make choices and these choices have consequences. Ask yourself which choices you are willing to live with and accept. To envy others is a distraction and waste of energy. Find your fit for the moment and accept what you are willing to live with and without.

Get a sense of what makes you feel alive, trust your intuition, and live life fully. When you live in this way your balanced energy ripples out and you inspire others to do the same. As we all know, there is no teacher like the teacher who teaches from example. With morality and introspection as your foundation, taking the right path is intuitive.

In short, *dharma* is the expression of your highest purpose in life. When you are living your dharma, you do not worry about what you should be doing. The ultimate beauty is that by living that which is most fulfilling to you, you are providing value to everyone who is impacted by your actions.

Moments of silence are essential to connect with your purpose. It's difficult (probably impossible) to reflect with shallow breath, it's difficult to reflect with an overactive mind, it's difficult to reflect when everything around us is noisy, and it's difficult to reflect when time slips away. Make space in your life, breathe deeply, hydrate, be quiet, and turn off any distractions and sounds (i.e., radio, television, etc.).

If you are caught up with what needs to be done, and have forgotten to ask what you want done, the following is a great place to start and get reacquainted with you.

For Reflection

Write everything that comes to mind when you ask yourself "who am I?" Then take aspects of what you wrote, and ask yourself where this label came from, whether it is serving you, and how attached you are to it. If it is not serving you, ask yourself whether you are willing to let it go. If the answer is no, ask why. If the answer is yes, ask when? Ask yourself what is it exactly that you want? And, where is it that you are going. What are you trying to achieve, have you "arrived"?

Artha

Recognized as the second aim of life. To live our purpose, having a place to live, clothes to wear, and the ability to be of service to humanity are well supported by wealth. *Artha* is also associated with the householder stage of our life. As young children, many of us did not worry about money; it was taken care of by the adults in our life. But then it becomes our turn, with many people finding themselves needing to provide for children, and also for ailing parents. Thus, part of your *dharma* becomes being of service to your family by providing financially.

Accumulating wealth just for the sake of accumulating wealth is not the purpose. Finding a balance takes reflection. Saving for rainy days without living in perpetual fear takes wisdom. Recognizing the impact that consumerism has on our environment, and making wise choices leads us in the right direction.

Also, there needs to be a connection with financial prosperity and the type of lifestyle that one wants to feel accomplished. My type of freedom is not your freedom. Acknowledging that prosperity is not about creating a life filled with wants and needs but that it's about knowing what is needed, and not overextend consumption, all while expressing gratitude leads us in a positive and balanced direction.

I was at a restaurant on a Saturday evening, and the woman working told me she hated the fact she had to work on a Saturday night. I told her I always felt prosperous for having a schedule that does not coincide with the majority. When I go grocery shopping, there is rarely a line up, I am hardly ever in traffic because I am going the other direction, and I can go cycling Tuesday mornings. She smiled, and to this day, feels grateful for the comment, and finds some peace in her irregular schedule. There is more than one way to look at a situation. Are you willing to expand your mind?

Without direction, chances are you will find yourself on a spinning wheel simply wanting more. The question is more of what, and at what cost. Prosperity is positive, a divine right, and blessing, but wealth at the expense of family, health, and quiet moments can actually become a big drain on our energy, and ability to be of service. There is a balance. Connecting with our centre allows each and every one to live it. Just like stretching our body – less is sometimes more.

For Reflection

How do you define prosperity? This is an individual definition. We all know that money is important, but what is it that you are going after? What is your freedom? What is your magic number? How important is it for you to compete with your neighbors? Why? How much time do you spend comparing yourself to others, or wishing you could buy this or that? What will this or that do for you? What are you willing to exchange for it? What type of lifestyle makes you feel alive? How many hours do you want to work? Stop and take a breath; you may realize that you do not really want what it is that you are chasing. The media may simply have convinced you that without it, you are incomplete.

Let your *artha* serve you and others. Use money for good – save and share. Enjoy it, but do not get too attached to it. The attachment could create resentment and fear; thus, eliminate the positive side of prosperity.

Kama

Relationships, human contact, and making space in your life for the people you love. In our lifetime, we will encounter many relationships, but one of the most important is the relationship the mind has with the body, because this foundation impacts the relationships we have with life itself.

An unhealthy relationship between mind and body includes having high expectations in terms of desired appearance often based on the media's definition of beauty. This is unhealthy for many obvious reasons. One of these reasons being that the body ages and changes, regardless of desires. Also, a total disconnect is unhealthy. Some people spend their entire life in their head, with the body being a tool to get the head from place to place. If something hurts it's quickly numbed with a drug; no questioning, no exploring, numb it, and move on.

A healthy mental relationship with the body can be defined as one of respect for the perfection of its individuality as well as for the mysteries of its magnificence. It's a loving relationship allowing the mind and the body to work together, nurturing a relationship of acceptance of its changes, and of the aging process. This also includes acceptance of what is, as it is. The grass is not always greener on the other side.

As for the relationship with the mind, take some time to be silent. Return to the beginning of your journal, review how the different aspects of your mind present themselves and pay attention.

Remember that wisdom is not the accumulation of intellectual facts, although heightened knowledge can be a source of great freedom, the wrong knowledge can be a source of more suffering and distraction. Therefore (trust me, I know), you do not need to run out and buy every spiritual book on the market, just sit for a moment and breathe.

The following is a statement from Swami Rama, founder of the Himalayan Institute in Pennsylvania, notably known as one of the first yogis to allow himself to be studied by western scientists. Scientists at the Menninger Clinic (a leading American inpatient psychiatric hospital) examined, and studied Rama's ability to voluntarily control bodily processes (i.e., heartbeat, blood pressure, body temperature, etc.) that are normally considered to be non-voluntary (autonomic). Regarding the mind, Rama says:

> *"The mind is the greatest of all mysteries. Upon unveiling this mystery, all mysteries are unveiled. The mind is the source of all misery and happiness. It is the source of both bondage and liberation. The more you know about your mind, the greater the mastery you will have over the world around you. The mind is an energy field. It is the finest manifestation of nature. Nature has deposited its entire bounty -all potentials, capacities and intelligence - in the mind. The mind is endowed with all creativity, imaginable and unimaginable. It has the capacity to create anything it wishes. It has enormous space to store its unlimited experiences and keep them as long as it likes."*

> (Yoga International, Summer 2011, p. 34.)

Every relationship we choose to cultivate has an impact on our *dharma*. Relationships can support or suppress our *dharma*, which is highly dependent on how the person's presence fits in with our belief system, and whether we react or respond to their energy. We must create a surplus of energy to be able to share it. Life consists of many little relationships all wrapped up into one, look for the similarities in your relationships. Write about what you see.

When we wake up to our thinking patterns, when we pay attention to our body language, we clearly see what we put out, therefore, releasing negative holding patterns. The relationship we have with ourselves ripples out.

For Reflection

What do you see first when you look at someone, do you see what they are wearing or their eyes? What type of relationships do you cultivate? Are you trustworthy; honest; reliable; attentive; caring; giving; needy; gossipy; or greedy? Where is the balance? How would your closest friends define you? Do you care about animals? Do you care about others you have never met? What is your relationship to life? What are your strengths? What are your weaknesses? Are you willing to grow? Are you willing to expand your perspectives?

In *sutra* 1.33, Patanjali introduces a method that is recognized throughout the world and it is also a technique to move beyond the mentioned obstacles. Patanjali states, "In relationships, the mind becomes purified by cultivating feelings of friendliness towards those who are happy, compassion for those who are suffering, goodwill towards those who are virtuous, and neutrality towards those we perceive as wicked or evil." This *sutra* becomes instrumental as we go through our own inner work, our life, who we believe we are, and how we project that belief. Sometimes I think, if I did nothing else but master this, my life would have great meaning. Being a part of this world means that we are always in action. Therefore, the actions that we take are beneficial to the whole when they support our inner truth.

For Reflection

Now let us reflect on the type of actions we can take to integrate and put this sutra in practice. Ask yourself, what is friendliness? Am I friendly? Am I a competitive person? Is this competitive nature a positive, and uplifting experience, or is it detrimental? Really think about this. It is possible to thrive and still be supportive of others. The attitude underlying the action is what has such an impact on its manifestation. Am I a jealous person? Does this jealousy prevent me from being friendly towards those who are happy or am I authentically friendly?

Having attended talks on dharma over the years, I have heard many masters kindly remind us that most of us have no friends because most of our relationships are conditional. It made me reflect on my friendships, and I can recall two separate and very meaningful events in my life where I really saw this truth. The first was when I was faced with a very challenging situation, where all of my friends started to disappear. I can also recall a time where something that is viewed as very positive happened and again, friends were less and less available. Jealousy can be a blinder. I started to look at my behavior to see what I needed to cultivate to be a true friend. I looked to see if I had been that person to others. What is important to you in friendship?

Who in this world does not prefer kindness over judgment? Who does not prefer a friend who can listen over a friend who always knows the answers? I see many people state that their favorite quote is Gandhi's "be the change you want to see in the world". Wonderful! Looks great on paper, sounds good out loud, but what type of actions are needed to be true to this?

How does compassion feel? Where does compassion arise from, and how does it manifest in your life? Who is virtuous? How would I offer goodwill? Perceptions of being wicked or evil – is it really a perception? Can I accept this? How does indifference present itself? Does this mean that I allow people to take advantage of others? If not, then how can I be indifferent and of service?

Kama is such a great place for practice for the urban practitioners as we are in continuous relationships. Remember to always review these words because as you clean your inner home, your mental clarity will improve, and as you start to nurture these qualities, you will be able to dive deeper.

We not only have relationships with ourselves and the people in our life, but inevitably, we have relationships with all of life. Nature itself surrounds us and is a part of us. The practice shows us that what we perceive outwardly is our inner projection: "*Yatha Brahmande Tadha Pindande*" (As within so without as without so within).

The *panca-bhuta*, which are the five elements of nature (earth, water, fire, air, and space) are a part of everything that surrounds us and of each other. Water is part of fire, and air is part of space, and so forth. Our bodies are a combination of the elements of earth, water, fire, air, and space. Each of our cells are made of each of these elements. Opening our eyes and seeing nature brings us in contact with this.

I love going to the ocean. Feeling the sand on my bare feet, connecting with the element of earth, the beauty, freshness and creativity of the water, the heat of the sun, the breeze caressing my skin, and the space and the vastness as I look at the sky, reminding me of the universe (no beginning, no end, always expanding). As within so without and as without so within. These same elements are a part of you.

Again, every day take some time and be with nature. Look at the sky, hug a tree, take a nature walk, and if you can, bathe in fresh water. If not, feel the snow, see and be with nature's bounty. Respect Mother Nature, walk softly on our planet (Remember that we are borrowing the planet from our children not inheriting it from our ancestors.).The more we connect with nature, the more we experience our interconnectedness with all of earth's creatures, increasing our potential for inner peace and compassion.

For Reflection

Do you make time for nature? Do you appreciate nature? Do you see nature? Do you crave the ocean or the mountains? What are you innately attracted to? Which aspects of nature take your breath away? Do you give yourself the time to be with nature? Do you look at the sky as you drive to work? Are you aware of the bounty that surrounds you? Can you appreciate a tree or a flower without needing to know what name we have given it? Do you need something different or can you appreciate what you have locally?

I have a family member who sees everything. When we go for a walk, you feel like you are with a child. She notices leaves, different blades of grass, and all the flowers, even the ones that blend in. We have a beautiful natural park near our home. I have a friend who lived in the area for 18 years before she visited the park. Work was always on her mind. What about you, where do you fit in? Can you take some time off? Write about nature, what you see and feel.

Now let us look at the power of sound and our relationship to it. Sound surrounds us at all times, and highly impacts our energy. Birds, wind, the sound of our own voice, which at times is musical and at other times is invasive, depending on where it is coming from and what we are speaking about. We have the sound of other people speaking, singing or yelling, traffic, construction and silence are all everyday examples. Recently I was at a *kirtan* (devotional singing), where a talented artist played many instruments. When he played the *esraj*, I instantly closed my eyes and felt the inner vibration of the instrument, which was beautiful and meditative. But then he played the drum, a beautiful instrument, but he was not as talented, and I instead felt an inner jarring as he pounded the drum. The more we open our ears to the sounds that surround us the more in tune we become with sound, and how it impacts us.

My daughter has always been someone who loves music. As young as five years old she would lie on the floor with headphones, and just listen to music. Many only listen to music in accordance with other activities, we like to have it as background sound as opposed to just listening to the music. Many feel uncomfortable with the silence of being home alone and put on the television or music to mask the intensity of the silence of listening to the inner sounds and thoughts vibrating within.

For Reflection

What is your relationship to sound, including your relationship to the most basic of sounds such as the sound of your own breath and the sound of your voice? Are you aware of how your voice changes and how its inner vibration impacts you and your world? Listen.

Try listening to music without doing anything else. Close your eyes and listen. Write about your experience. Listen to the sound of your voice as you speak. What are you saying? Where is your voice coming from? When we speak out of fear, or anger it often comes from the throat, and it is "non-impacting". When we speak our truth, the voice comes from our centre of gravity, it comes from the navel. Notice your voice, do you ever speak in a child-like voice, wanting to be nice, or are you aggressive? Listen for it.

Write about your voice. Write how you feel about the sound of your voice, the power of your voice, and where you feel it is coming from under different circumstances. Do people enjoy your voice? What type of energy does your voice carry? Be aware of how the sounds in your home impact your energy. We are such creatures of habit that we often sustain energy because it's habitual regardless of its impact. Enjoy the process.

Moksha

Liberation. Anything we say or write about liberation is not it because it cannot be conceptualized. With that said, liberation is often defined as a shift in consciousness that happens when we stop identifying as separate; it is a direct experience of "oneness". Referred to in Sanskrit as *sat* (truth), *chit* (as pure consciousness), and *ananada* (bliss as an experience beyond sensation), *moksha* is a direct experience beyond ordinary language that is limited by individual perceptions.

Although teachers and gurus are ideal and often essential on the path to growth, if we continuously read and listen to others sharing their experience of liberation, we make concepts of what we think their experiences are and then try to achieve that state, which can lead to disillusion and confusion. If, on the other hand, we have the privilege of encountering a guru, who can open us up to the experience of oneness instantly through transmission then the experience may trigger a deeper experience of life, or it may lead us still to an external search by depending on the guru for the returning experience.

We can, as the wise philosophers, and masters teach, live our life horizontally, which is characterized by extroversion, being preoccupied, or even obsessed at times with the external aspects of life such as consuming, socializing, ones status in life and such becoming life itself. When we live this way we accumulate things and experiences, but we often identify with them and relate to them as we always have, thus, preventing further inner growth. Living this way often means that how we relate to the world at 25 is how we relate to the world at 45.

Reflecting on *moksha* starts to resemble a more integral approach to life. From the perspective of *purushasartha* (purpose/fulfillment of life), as we age we have more free time and more opportunities for introspection. These moments of introspection, of meditation, of journaling, reading, and inquiry into our nature and of our life are what provide growth. In our materialistic world, however, we need to go out of our way to give this aspect some life as our culture does not seem to support it.

There are a variety of techniques to tap into the experience and hatha yoga is one of them. Hatha yoga is a tool for *moksha*. However, with hatha yoga's mass promotion and popularity of physical postures without meditation, breathing techniques, ethical lifestyles, and introspection, what we call yoga today has in some cases become another tool to support our neurosis, creating more bondage to the body and illusions of separateness, keeping us stuck in old fearful thinking.

Yoga was not designed to lead to obsessions about our body; it is not a tool to create separation by identifying with one methodology through the resentment or judgment of another. *Asanas* bring life, vitality, and energy to the body and mind, creating space and providing comfort for a happy and liberated life. Your body is a vehicle for your journey, let it be of service to you.

If you are a modern-day yogi(ni), and practice *asana* regularly, ask yourself what your yoga is doing for you. Many begin yoga asana to reduce back pain, improve sleep, or support sporting activities. Hatha yoga proves to be of service, but if we continue approaching our practice from this place, we may limit ourselves from the full experience and find ourselves in the perpetual cycle of wanting more of something whether it be flexibility, strength, beauty, or any other external desires that keep us identified with our small ego. If you have a regular *asana* practice, keep up, but also keep an open mind. Be aware of the attitude you cultivate towards your practice, the relationship you nurture on the mat and the thoughts you entertain as they are a reflection of your life off the mat. Open up to your practice fully, use your body as a tool for observation, give yourself some space to be receptive to the natural flow of nature. Meditate, there is no such thing as a bad meditation. Every moment counts. Meditation is a gift that just keeps on giving.

Another important aspect for *moksha* is the acceptance of death. If you ask some people if they are prepared for death what is often understood by this question is whether one's finances are in order. To expand on our preparation for death, reflecting on its certainty and yet uncertainty is a powerful technique for *moksha*. Facing our mortality can wake us up to life. The reflection helps to lessen worries and anger. It opens our heart and reminds us that everyone is dying and facing the same uncertainty. This acceptance frees us little by little from the bondage of the mind that creates fear and separation.

It's easier to ignore our death in our youth than it is in our golden years because our golden years are a reflection of death arriving. Always remember that it's not negative to reflect on death, it is actually quite the opposite – greed is reduced, nit-picking is reduced, beauty and appreciation are increased. However, don't take my word for it. Reflect.

Depending on where you are in your life, age, and situation, you may be required to focus more on one of the aims of life. You may be in need of money to support your family, or you may be at a time where you can focus on spirituality.

What is valuable is seeing where you are, what your strengths are, and what could be cultivated. For example, you love your work, you are doing exactly what you want to do, and you are making a meaningful wage. Beautiful! If you are still feeling unsettled look outside of the money and purpose realms.

For Reflection

Remind yourself of the choices you have made and the life you are living. Each and everyone's starting point is unique, and our relationship to our starting point can be of service, or it can be a detriment. Look – really look – at the vastness of the sky, no beginning and no end, continuously expanding. And now ask yourself again: Who am I? What do I want? Where am I going?

"A man should look for what is, and not for what he thinks should be."
Albert Einstein

Chapter 12

Gratitude

Over dinner one evening, a friend was telling us how grateful he is about life. The life force in his voice, the sparkle in his eyes, the bounce in his step are proof that he really feels this. After a near death experience, he says he wakes up every morning with the desire to express gratitude for life itself. I too found my gratitude voice and heart in hardship, but I now feel it fully and have learned to maintain it, nourish it, and fuel it with life itself. By expressing gratitude with intention, we can breathe life into the action and the results are a tangible experience.

It is my understanding that the study and the science of gratitude are relatively new. What I find interesting is the desire for some to see the science before engaging in the practice. Gratitude is the type of thing that is priceless and requires very little time. By developing the habit consciously, not mechanically, we create internal shifts and respond to life with appreciation as opposed to reacting with fear. Instead of looking outside ourselves for the science, we live it regardless of what is said and whom says it.

I spent some time recently with someone who has a strong belief about life being cruel and out to get her. It was interesting to observe and see how whatever situation we were in, she was always looking for the negative, looking to prove her point, and justify her belief system. We are all on some level doing the same thing. We try to justify our point of view and look for examples that support it. Which point of view are you trying to prove?

My daughter was going through a challenging time with lots on her mind such as school, work, gym, friends, etc. How do I balance it all? We had some great chats, finding balance, and releasing tension. Then I sent her an email asking her to write five things she was grateful for. I told her she could not just think about it, or ignore this email, she had to do it.

The reply I received was confirmation of the impact this powerful technique plays in our life. I could feel how she had relaxed and could see with more clarity what needed to be done to reconnect with her centre of balance and let it ripple out, rather than trying to build it from the outside in.

For me, journaling as introspection can at times be challenging. I do not always feel like being honest or mindful about my path or my thoughts, at times I just want to forget about it and live mechanically. However, I am committed to keeping a journal. Expressing gratitude is such a great way to stay connected with writing and with what is important in life. It helps us remember what we value and why we value it. One of the things I am eternally grateful for is the fact that I care about growth and spirituality. I cannot imagine living without either and often express gratitude for having the stamina to show up.

I know from experience that it is easier to keep up than to start over. I express gratitude for everything, health, human contact, love, human rights, the sun, fresh and abundant food supplies, my eyesight...the list goes on. I am also grateful when I experience difficult times. I am grateful for the learning opportunities, for having the tools and understanding to move beyond them, and for the experience of life as a whole.

In this section, write what you are grateful for. Write full sentences such as, I am grateful for having the energy and time to journal, rather than writing, "journaling". Remember to date your entries and to review what you write. As you will experience, the revision is proof of the internal shifts that happen because you will read about limiting beliefs you no longer live by and you will see how the quality of your introspection changes.

We are often told to live in the now, to be present, but this has the potential of remaining conceptual if it is done through the lens of the mind gaining knowledge and making concepts of now. What we aim for is a seeing beyond concept. Time as we know it is an illusion and the experience yogi's are leading us toward is beyond time and space as the mind understands it. The more you write, the more you will see your mind at play. The observation creates a distance between the seer and the seen, leading to inner peace, clarity, and trust in the process of life. With the conscious habits you have created, as well as with the willingness to live morally, you reduce your negative karmic imprints and establish a relationship with your centre of equanimity. What could be better? Visit this section often. It does not take much time or even much energy. Yet it provides you with so much in return and reminds us of what is important in life. Remember how short it is and choose to be the light and a source of inspiration for yourself.

> *"Do you know my attitude? Books, scriptures,*
> *and things like that only point out the way to reach*
> *God. After finding the way, what more need is there*
> *of books and scriptures? Then comes the time for*
> *action."*
>
> Ramakrishna

Chapter 13   **Affirmations**

There is a verse attributed to the *Upanishads* that states:

> *Watch your thoughts; they become words.*
> *Watch your words; they become actions.*
> *Watch your actions; They become habits.*
> *Watch your habits for they form your character.*
> *Watch your character as it determines your destiny.*

It's not uncommon to use affirmations in the following manner: I am ready to meet the partner of my choice; I deserve to make x dollars yearly; or I am the winner of the race, and so forth. If one is wanting a partner to the point that this is all she sees and thinks about, think of the beauty she misses around her, spending most conversations with friends trying to figure out how to attract the right person and why it has not happened. Really, what we are all after is happiness, and we cannot put a price on happiness, nor can we say, "Once I have this, that and this then I will be happy." Happiness is now, as it is.

What I am offering is to use affirmations as a tool to remind yourself of the natural beauty and perfection that lies within, instead of focusing on the expected outward desire. As we connect with our centre, our overall energy and communication with life changes, thus attracting what is in line with our unique path.

Choose one of the following affirmations and write it out 108 times per day for the next 120 days. Then, if you choose, you can change affirmations. You can also use these affirmations to direct the mind away from continuous mental chatter by mentally repeating them as you go about your daily life. Apparently, most of the things we think about, we think about most of the time. Therefore, if we spend a few minutes a day consciously moving away from this spiral, we will not miss anything.

The affirmations are:

    Aham Samatva – Balance, equanimity is my true nature;
    Aham Santosham – Contentment is my true nature;
    Aham Shanti – Peace is my true nature; and
    Aham Ananda – Bliss is my true nature.

Writing them in Sanskrit imprints the subconscious with truth and reduces the potential for an unconscious negating of the affirmation. Also, we want to avoid creating an expectation of a desired outcome. If we use the aspect of the mind that is scattered to determine what we believe we are after we end up chasing a fantasy. Concentrate and write it out with care. Remember also that the benefit of one of these affirmations is the realization and experience of all of them.

Choose an affirmation you are drawn to and with discipline, concentration, respect and patience explore it daily. This practice can be done anytime and anywhere. What is important is the commitment. Having faith in the process and moving beyond the obstacles that may arise.

Sutra 1.36, also provides us with an antidote for the obstacles listed in chapter 3. Patanjali tells us that contemplating the luminous light arising from the heart centre brings peace of mind. To help with this, keeping our awareness at the heart centre, front and back, and inhaling "A" and exhaling 'Ham' and then vibrating *santosham* at the heart centre supports this experience. I recommend practising this five minutes in the morning and five minutes at night.

> *"Yoga is possible for anybody who really wants it.*
> *Yoga is universal…. But don't approach yoga with a*
> *business mind looking for worldly gain."*
> Pathabis Jois

Chapter 14

Free Flow

Here you write about how you feel in the moment: joy, sadness, conversations, dreams, and your personal interpretation of your dreams.

For example, imagine that your life is going very well, you and your family are healthy, you are loved, able to love, you have freedom, enjoy your work, and so forth. But, you have sorrow due to a relationship that has caused you stress and are unable to let it go.

You would write something like this: What I am attached to? Why am I still pained by this? Can I forgive this person? Why? When? How would I feel if I was to let it go? Continue to ask yourself questions, you will be pleased to see the wisdom that resides in you.

Trust your intuition. Write about what you need to get off your chest and also write about what you would like to remember. Think of yourself 10 years your senior reading today's story. Bring a smile to your future lips.

"Insanity: doing the same thing over and over again
and expecting different results."
Albert Einstein

Chapter 15

Progress Report

As you read over your thoughts and review your belief systems, you will see how they change. Write about what has changed and the progress you see in yourself when you read your journal. For example, you may notice that your definition of patience has changed because you feel integrated with the experience of patience in contrast to trying to be patient. Write about how this feels and looks in your life. Also write about what has not changed. Why has it not? Where is the blockage coming from? Is it a conscious or unconscious choice?

In closing, I remind you to keep writing and to keep reviewing your writing. Be kind and honest with yourself. Observe, keep up and always let go. Experience the benefits of self awareness by keeping a log of your life and how you experience your life. Be as creative as you like, add chapters if you feel drawn to it, pictures, poems, quotes, but let the creative expression come from you. This is your journal, your journey, your exploration. The beauty is that it does lead to mutual growth because as you awaken to your inner beauty the ripple effect impacts those around you.

"May we be blessed with the courage to always keep up and the wisdom to always let go."
OM Shanti. Sylvie

Bibliography

Distance-Learning Course Classical Yoga. Georg Feuerstein. Eastend: Traditional Yoga Studies, 2008.

Bhagavad Gita and Its Message. Sri Aurobindo. Twin Lakes: Lotus Press, 1995.

The Bhagavad Gita. Swami Sivananda. Tehri-Garhwal: The Divine Life Society, 2003.

Bliss Divine. Swami Sivananda. Tehri-Garhwal: The Divine Life Society, 2004.

Deeper Dimensions of Yoga. Georg Feuerstein. Boston: Shambhala Publications, 1997.

Essence of Principal Upanishads. Swami Sivananda. Tehri-Garhwal: The Divine Life Society, 1998.

The Hatha Yoga Pradipika. Brian Dana Akers. Woodstock: YogaVidya.com, 2002.

Hatha Yoga Pradipika. Swami Muktibodhananda. Munger: Yoga Publications Trust, 1998.

The Hatha Yoga Pradipika. Vishnu Devananda. New Delhi: Motilal Banarsidass Publishers, 1987.

The Integral Yoga. Sri Aurobindo. Pondicherry: Sri Aurobindo Ashram Press, 1993.

Living Tantra Seminars. Pandit Rajmani Tigunait. Honesdale: Himalayan Institute, 2011-2012.

Mantra Yoga and Primal Sound: Secrets of Seed. David Frawley. Twin Lakes: Lotus Press, 2010.

The Philosophical and Religious Lectures of Swami Vivekananda. Swami Tapasyananda. Location: Advaita Ashrama, 1984.

Powers Within. Sri Aurobindo and The Mother. Twin Lakes: Lotus Press, 1998.

Ramana, Shankara and the Forty Verses Alan Jacobs. London: Watkins Publishing, 2002.

The Shambhala Encyclopedia of Yoga. Georg Feuerstein. Boston: Shambhala Publications, 1997.

Vedantic Meditation: Lighting the Flame of Awareness. David Frawley. Berkeley: North Atlantic Books, 2000.

The Yoga-Sutras of Patanjali: A New Translation and Commentary. Georg Feuerstein. Rochester: Inner Traditions Bear & Company, 1989.

CPSIA information can be obtained at www.ICGtesting.com
Printed in the USA
LVOW012205020413

327252LV00027B/1244/P

9 781770 842670